BLUENOSE *Bluebirds*

NOVA SCOTIA'S MILITARY NURSES IN THE GREAT WAR

Brian Douglas Tennyson

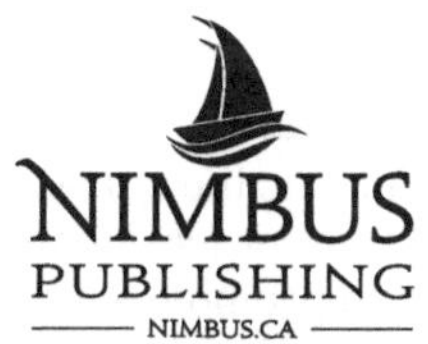

Nimbus Publishing Limited
3660 Strawberry Hill Street, Halifax, NS, B3K 5A9
(902) 455-4286 nimbus.ca

Nimbus Publishing is based in Kjipuktuk, Mi'kma'ki, the traditional territory of the Mi'kmaq People.

Printed and bound in Canada
NB 1859

Editor: Raya Morrison
Editor for the press: Angela Mombourquette
Interior design: Bee Stanton
Cover design: Heather Bryan

Cover images: Above: Margaret Macdonald. [Canadian Nurses Association/Library and Archives Canada/e003525007]. Below: Nursing sisters in front of the matron's tent at the Canadian Army Medical Corps. Canadian Stationary Hospital, no. 7, in Arques, France. [Dal Archives, PC1, Box 63, Folder 37]

Library and Archives Canada Cataloguing in Publication

Title: Bluenose bluebirds : Nova Scotia's military nurses in the Great War / Brian Douglas Tennyson.

Names: Tennyson, Brian Douglas, author

Description: Includes bibliographical references and index.

Identifiers: Canadiana (print) 20250331942 | Canadiana (ebook) 20250333007 | ISBN 9781774715178 (softcover) | ISBN 9781774715185 (EPUB)

Subjects: LCSH: Nurses—Nova Scotia—Biography. | LCSH: Nurses—Nova Scotia—History—20th century. | LCSH: Military nursing—Nova Scotia—History—20th century. | LCSH: World War, 1914-1918—Nova Scotia—Biography. | LCSH: World War, 1914-1918—Medical care—Nova Scotia. | LCSH: World War, 1914-1918—Women—Nova Scotia. | LCSH: Nova Scotia—Biography. | LCGFT: Biographies. | LCGFT: Informational works.

Classification: LCC D629.C2 T46 2026 | DDC 940.4/757160922—dc23

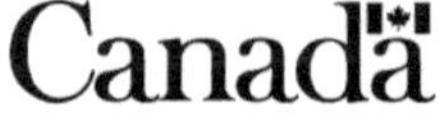

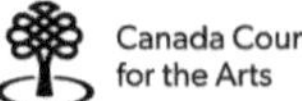

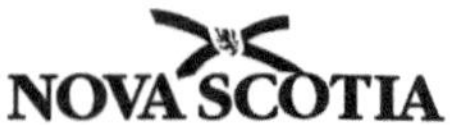

Nimbus Publishing acknowledges the financial support for its publishing activities from the Government of Canada, the Canada Council for the Arts, and from the Province of Nova Scotia. We are pleased to work in partnership with the Province of Nova Scotia to develop and promote our creative industries for the benefit of all Nova Scotians.

In remembrance of Sandy
and dedicated to Lindsay
my favourite nurse

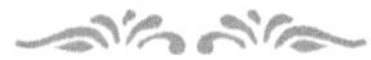

No. 1 Canadian General Hospital Nursing Sisters' Theme*

In my sweet little Alice Blue gown
When I first came to Birmingham town,
I had a bad trip, in a nasty old ship
And the cold in my billet just gave me the pip.
We came out to nurse our own troops
But were greeted with measles and whoop
Now I'll be a granny
*And keep warm with turpentine stupes.***
In my sweet little Alice Blue gown,
When I return to my home town
They will bring out the band, give the girls a big hand.
Being a nurse in the force, I'll be quite renowned
And I'll never forget all the fun
That I had, since I joined Number One.
*I was happy and gay, to have served with MacRae****
In my sweet little Alice Blue gown.

---

* No. 1 Canadian General Hospital was organized at Valcartier on September 14, 1914, from the active militia unit, No. 5 Field Ambulance, of Montreal.

** A piece of soft cloth or absorbent cotton, dipped in hot water and used to make a poultice.

*** "MacRae" obviously refers to John McCrae; he served in No. 3 Canadian General Hospital, not No. 1 Canadian General Hospital.

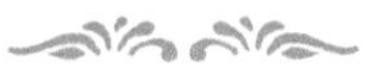

Contents

Preface

In 2017 I published a book entitled *Nova Scotia at War, 1914–1919*, the first attempt to tell the story of the province's experience of the First World War. That led me to determine how many Nova Scotian soldiers served in the war, the military units in which they served, their experiences, and how many of them lost their lives. I included military nurses, of course, but didn't give them the attention that I came to realize they deserved. This book grew out of that.

Somewhat to my surprise, it appeared that very little has been written about Canadian military nurses in the war. There is, in fact, just one book that tells their story: *Sister Soldiers of the Great War: The Nurses of the Canadian Army Medical Corps*, written by Cynthia Toman and published in 2016. It built on Susan Mann's excellent biography, *Margaret Macdonald: Imperial Daughter*, published in 2005. Macdonald was the matron-in-chief of the Canadian Army Medical Corps Nursing Service (CAMCNS). Having said that, I soon discovered the many memoirs, diaries, biographies and magazine articles written by or about Canadian (including Newfoundland) military nurses who served in the First World War.

Margaret Macdonald was a Nova Scotian, and that led me to wonder how many Nova Scotian nurses served in the war. This book is the result. It tells not only how many Nova Scotian nurses served in the war and who they were, but also their experiences in the war and their lives before and after.

This has not been a simple matter because, more than a century later, historians still don't agree on how many Canadian military nurses served in the war. What is generally agreed is that half of all Canadian doctors and between a third and a half of nurses served in uniform in the war.[1] Veterans Affairs Canada cautiously claims only that "more than 2,800" served in the CAMCNS[2], while Colonel J. G. Adami's figure was 2,428, and Macdonald's own estimate was 2,951, although in 1922 she raised that number to 3,141 by including 190 Queen Alexandra's Imperial Military Nursing Service (QAIMNS) nurses.[3] Toman concluded that the precise number was 2,845 and Nova Scotia provided the second highest number of nurses based on place of birth: 250 (12.1%), compared to Ontario's 1,189 (57.5%).[4] Only 2,816 of them were fully trained nurses, however, because several women served in auxiliary roles that supported the nurses, 2,504 of whom served in England, France and the eastern Mediterranean.[5]

The key point is that both Veterans Affairs Canada and Toman only included nurses who served in the CAMCNS alongside the more than 600,000 soldiers whose service records are available in the Veterans Affairs Canada database. That was significant because, unlike the military nurses of other countries—notably QAIMNS, the nursing service of the British army—they were officers in the Canadian army, which meant that they were well paid but the army had control "not only over their behaviour and activities as women in the all-male domain of war but also over their movements and postings."[6] It is not known how many Canadian nurses served in the QAIMNS because its records are not accessible. Its requirements were similar to those of the CAMCNS, however, and the QAIMNS actively recruited Canadian nurses in nursing journals, nursing association magazines and even newspapers, and at least 313 Canadian and Newfoundland nurses are thought to have served in it.[7]

Many of these women may have come from families that had emigrated in recent years and understandably turned to their mother country in its time of need. They may also have been attracted to serving in an auxiliary voluntary organization led by the Queen of England, but "at least 18" of them subsequently transferred into the CAMCNS, where they were actual army officers and were paid more than QAIMNS nurses. Unfortunately, only 9 (Frances Cron, Elsie Doyle, Bertha Forsey, Frances Maitland Frew, Grace Gardner, Isabel Holden, Martha Loder, Maysie Parsons and Katherine White) have been identified.

Toman only included QAIMNS nurses if they served overseas, but I include Nova Scotians who were among the 447 nurses who served in military hospitals in Canada and Newfoundland.[8] That complicates the situation because many of them served overseas before or after their QAIMNS service.[9] Similarly, Toman included an unknown number of nurses who had trained in the United States and joined the United States Army Corps or medical units formed by American universities to support the British and French medical services. One was the surgery unit created by Harvard University, the Massachusetts General Hospital and two other hospitals, which went overseas in March 1915 under the auspices of the Red Cross to provide staffing at the American Ambulance Hospital in Paris. By November 1916 its members were functioning as members with commissioned rank in the Royal Army Medical Corps and were stationed at the RAMC No. 22 General Hospital at Camiers.

Eighteen Nova Scotian nurses who had trained in the northeastern states—Vera Benjamin, Emily Brennan, Frieda Christie, Eva Clements, Marguerite Condon, Bertha Cray, Evangeline Eaton, Lillian Edgecombe, Marion Ellis, Ethel Etherington, Lydia Ferguson, Marguerite Gray, Harriett Harlow, Hazel King, Dorothea MacInnis, Marion MacLeod, Ann Murray and Katharine Van Buskirk—served in it, and some subsequently transferred into the CAMCNS.

Similarly, at least eight Canadian nurses sponsored by the Canadian National Association of Trained Nurses (CNATN) were sent to England in 1915 in response to an appeal from the French Flag Nursing Corps, a British organization that provided British, Irish and Commonwealth nurses to the Société Française de Secours aux Blessés Militaires—the French Red Cross—to the French army.[10] I do not include women who served in voluntary nursing organizations such as the St. John Ambulance Association's Voluntary Aid Detachment

(VAD) because very few of them were professional nurses, although I do discuss the significant role they played in supporting nurses in hospitals overseas and at home.[11]

I also include a handful of Nova Scotian nurses who made significant contributions overseas through international refugee organizations and two women who served overseas in the Société Française de Secours aux Blessés Militaires because one was a trained nurse and the other's experience provides a broader understanding of Nova Scotia's role in the war, both overseas and at home.

After the war some nurses left Nova Scotia because they married men they had met during the war, and others moved elsewhere because Nova Scotia's economy slumped badly after the war. That didn't affect nurses as much as it did women who had entered the wartime workforce, however, because there were more hospitals than before the war, although there were also more nurses seeking employment. Some sought to remain in the CAMC—renamed the Royal Canadian Army Medical Corps in 1920—but that was not really an option because the postwar army slashed the nursing service to just twelve personnel. Many nurses wisely retrained for emerging professions in social work, public health, school and frontier nursing, and physiotherapy, and some simply retired.[12]

All Canadian nurses who served in the war merit recognition for their service, but Nova Scotia's military nurses were different because their province was the only one in Canada that was directly exposed to the war. Both Halifax and Sydney were defended ports from which Canadian and American convoys carried vital cargoes to Britain while being attacked by German submarines. Halifax was also a major Canadian point of departure for soldiers and the reception point for most of the wounded men being brought home for convalescent medical treatment.[13] It was also, of course, the only community in Canada that experienced massive destruction and loss of life due to the war when two ships collided in its harbour in December 1917.

One nurse who doesn't really qualify in this book, but I think should be recognized, is Alice Margaret Blood, who was born in

England and didn't move to Canada until 1920. I include her because she had trained at St. Bartholomew's Hospital in London, joined the QAIMNS and served in No. 16 Canadian General Hospital at Orpington, England. There she met a Nova Scotian physician, Dr. Hugh MacKinnon, who was from East Lake Ainslie, Inverness County. They fell in love and, after returning to Canada in July 1919, they married and over the years lived in Inverness, Berwick, and Halifax. Obviously, Blood does not qualify as a Bluenose Bluebird, but she did become a Nova Scotian and spent the rest of her life there. She was, I believe, the last surviving Nova Scotian military nurse from the First World War when she died at the age of 105 in the Camp Hill Veterans Memorial wing of the Queen Elizabeth II Health Sciences Centre in 1999.

This raises the question of who should be considered a Nova Scotian. Most were born there, others moved there for various reasons, and, of course, many moved elsewhere. I, for example, was not born in Nova Scotia but have lived and worked there for most of my life and consider myself a Nova Scotian. I therefore include not only nurses who were born in Nova Scotia, but also those who moved there for various reasons, perhaps because their families did or to attend one of the province's two nursing schools, and decided to stay.

This largely explains why my database has 311 entries instead of Toman's 250. The number of entries in the database is slightly skewed because 14 of them are cross-references reflecting name changes, so my actual number of entries is 297.

Readers should be aware that some confusion may occur with names beginning with "Mac" or "Mc" because the spelling was often inconsistent, even within families. I have used the spelling used by the nurses themselves, regardless of how others, including relatives, spelled their name. Similarly, those who have examined the service records of nurses will have noticed that they appear to have served in the CAMC Depot at Shorncliffe in addition to the medical units in which they served. This is misleading because nurses did not actually serve in the depot; all Canadian military nurses were carried on its roll on their arrival in England before being posted to CAMC units or were there while temporarily unfit or awaiting discharge.

This book is divided into two sections. The first briefly tells the stories of Nova Scotia's military nurses as revealed in their letters, diaries, memoirs and biographies, including coping with the horrors of modern war and death on a scale that they could not have imagined.[14] Those who served in military and civilian hospitals in Nova Scotia and elsewhere also found themselves having to cope with the influenza pandemic, the greatest global epidemic in modern history. The second part is a database that lists all Nova Scotian nurses who served in the war that I could identify and includes brief biographies not only of their wartime experience but also as much as possible of their pre-war and postwar lives. Even so, it has not been possible to find much information about a few of them.

The primary sources for the information contained in this book are the personnel records of the First World War database at Library and Archives Canada, the Canadian Virtual War Memorial, and the genealogy records of the Nova Scotia Archives, all of which are available online. I have made extensive use of census records and the wealth of information available on Ancestry.com but also conducted many random internet searches that were often very helpful and enhanced the life stories of these women. I have also read every relevant book, journal article and postgraduate dissertation that I could find, and they are listed in the lengthy bibliography.

Finally, I am profoundly grateful to those who have shared their research with me or helped with this project in other ways. Wendy Robichaud, archivist at Acadia University, generously shared her information on women who had attended Acadia's Ladies' Seminary before training at nursing schools. William Jones, historic archives specialist at the McGill University Health Centre, went above and beyond to enable me to be the first historian to identify one of the nurses who served at the Royal Canadian Naval Hospital at the time of the Halifax explosion. Dr. Heidi Coombs and Professor Terry Bishop Stirling of Memorial University generously helped me sort out which units Newfoundland nurses served in. And, once again I am indebted to Anna MacNeil, archival research assistant at Cape Breton University's Beaton Institute, and Mary Campbell and Amanda McNeil, CBU's library technicians, who kindly sent me copies of important but not readily available books. Mitchell Jabalee, CBU's library technician for special collections and circulation, even promptly corrected a page reference for me!

In my research I discovered, much to my surprise, that Gloria (Webb) Stephens, a retired Nova Scotian nurse, had privately published *Remembering Nurses Who Served* in 2020. It only tells the stories of nurses who trained at Halifax's Victoria General Hospital but includes those who served not only in the First World War but also the Second World War, Korea, and Vietnam. A labour of love, it provides much useful information and many photographs but unfortunately is sometimes seriously unreliable and is not readily available in libraries.

Once again, I am grateful to my late wife, Sandra Atwell-Tennyson, who as always encouraged this project, correcting awkward sentences, misspellings, and errors, but did not live to see the completed book. Luckily, Angela Mombourquette, Nimbus' adult non-fiction editor, brought in Raya P. Morrison, who proved to be an empathic assistant who improved the final text. Any errors that may have slipped through are, of course, entirely mine.

Brian Douglas Tennyson
Bedford, Nova Scotia
July 23, 2025

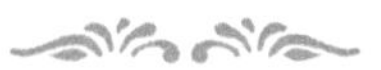

Glossary

CAMC	Canadian Army Medical Corps
CAMCNS	Canadian Army Medical Corps Nursing Service
CANSR	Canadian Army Nursing Service Reserve
CCC	CAMC Casualty Company
CCCS	Canadian Casualty Clearing Station
CEF	Canadian Expeditionary Force
CGH	Canadian General Hospital
CSH	Canadian Stationary Hospital
CHH	Camp Hill Hospital, Halifax
CMH	Cogswell Street Military Hospital, Halifax
DCRC	Duchess of Connaught Canadian Red Cross Hospital
MD	Military District
MGH	Montreal General Hospital
NGH	Newfoundland General Hospital
PAMC	Permanent Active Militia Medical Corps
QAIMNS	Queen Alexandra's Imperial Military Nursing Service
RDS	Rockhead Infectious Diseases Hospital
RMC	Rockhead Military Hospital
RAMC	Royal Army Medical Corps
RNH	Royal Canadian Naval Hospital
RVH	Royal Victoria Hospital, Montreal
SFSBM	Société Française de Secours aux Blessés Militaires
SJAA	St. John Ambulance Association
SOS	Struck off service
TFNS	Territorial Force Nursing Service
VAD	Voluntary Aid Detachment
VGH	Victoria General Hospital, Halifax

Introduction

When Britain declared war on Germany in August 1914, the Canadian parliament promptly declared its support and began recruiting volunteers for overseas service. The Canadian army—or "permanent force" as it was called—consisted of only about 3,100 personnel, an unimpressive number but one that seemed adequate because it was only intended to form the nucleus of a much larger force that would be raised from the militia, which had about 43,000 personnel in 1914.

The army was a much more sophisticated and complex organization than it had been in the South African War because the government of Sir Wilfrid Laurier—under the leadership of Sir Frederick Borden, the long-term minister of militia—had introduced major reforms that made the army a much more professional organization than what it had been in the South African War. In 1904 the inadequate practice of employing physicians in each of the military districts and contracting civilian nurses only when needed was replaced by the Permanent Active Militia Medical Corps (PAMC), while the militia component became the Army Medical Corps (AMC).

The PAMC included physicians and support staff but also nurses, who were required to be female and were given the rank and pay of officers, a remarkably progressive—and practical—decision that aroused stiff resistance in some circles and did not reflect British policy.[15] In 1909 the PAMC and AMC were merged into the Canadian Army Medical Corps (CAMC).

A year later the Canadian Army Nursing Reserve (CANSR) was created, as well, for civilian female nurses between twenty-three and forty-five years of age who agreed to serve for five years. If they served in Canada, they were under the regulations of the CAMC, but if they served elsewhere in the empire, they were under the regulations of Queen Alexandra's Imperial Military Nursing Service (QAIMNS), the British army's nursing service. They completed a one-month military nursing course and annual training camps at the new Cogswell Street Military Hospital (CMH) in Halifax, which was close to the Halifax garrison and the naval base. That made them eligible to join the CAMC Nursing Service (CAMCNS) if there were vacancies or be posted to hospitals and similar institutions.[16]

The PAMC had only two nurses when it was created: Georgina Fane Pope and Margaret Clotilde Macdonald. Pope was a daughter of William Pope, a Prince Edward Island Father of Confederation, a niece of James Pope, who had been premier in 1865–67, 1870–72 and 1873, and sister of Sir Joseph Pope, who had been John A. Macdonald's private secretary and later served as deputy minister of the Department of External Affairs from 1896 to 1926 under the prime minister. After graduating from the New York School for Nurses at Bellevue Hospital, Pope was superintendent of the Columbia Hospital for Women in Washington, DC, where she founded a school of nursing, then was superintendent of St. John's Riverside Hospital in Yonkers, New York. In 1899 she was appointed senior sister in charge of the Canadian nurses in the South African War.

Macdonald was a graduate of the New York City Charity Hospital School for Nurses and had an impressive record of overseas service in the Spanish-American War and the South African War and had served for eighteen months with the Health Department of the US in the Canal Zone when the Panama Canal was under construction.[17]

In 1908 Pope and Macdonald were both posted to Halifax, where Pope served as the first matron of the Cogswell Street Military Hospital (CMH), which was close to the Wellington Barracks, and both trained civilian nurses for military service in case of war.[18] When the war broke out, however, Pope was not appointed matron-in-chief of the CAMCNS because of her age—she was fifty-two—and Macdonald was appointed instead. She was also over age but much younger than Pope. Both, therefore, set a precedent that many nurses followed when they joined the CAMCNS because they were rarely required to provide proof of their date of birth or, on the whole, of anything else that they claimed. To her credit, Pope subsequently signed up for overseas service in August 1917 and was serving in No. 2 Canadian Stationary Hospital (CSH) at Outreau when it was bombed in May 1918. She was not wounded but suffered neurasthenia and returned home in December 1918.[19]

Macdonald proved to be a good choice for matron-in-chief because she essentially had to create the position and develop policies and regulations for what became a large and complex organization. She was not autonomous, however, because she was directly answerable to Major General Guy Carleton Jones,[20] a Nova Scotian physician who was the CEF's director of medical services. He came under the "overall nursing authority" of Maud McCarthy, who was not only the matron-in-chief of the QAIMNS but also had "overall responsibility" for all British and Commonwealth nurses "in France and Flanders."[21]

When the war broke out in August 1914, there were only five CAMCNS nurses, fifty-seven nurses in the militia,[22] and a small reserve of civilian nurses who had completed a one-month military nursing course or attended a brief military nursing training camp or both. More nurses than that were going to be required and more than one thousand volunteered in 1914. That was significant because, as historian Susan Mann has pointed out, "there were always more applicants than places" and "with graduate nurses increasing in number, the war offered an unusual opportunity."[23]

Most of the young nurses who initially joined the CAMCNS had no military experience but, as historian Gillian Woodford points out, they found themselves "returning to the residential, uniformed, disciplined, hierarchical life of school and hospital" while being given officer status in the army and receiving better pay than they could earn in civilian nursing. That meant that they could focus on actual nursing because most of their non-nursing duties would be taken care of by male orderlies or female volunteers, although "some of the younger lower-ranked men...balked at having to take orders from women."[24] Even so, they were "embarking on an unusual adventure for women" and "intended to make the most of it."[25]

In order to qualify, they were required to be British subjects, Caucasian, between twenty-one and thirty-eight years of age, unmarried or widowed, possessing high moral character and dignified deportment, and graduates of recognized three-year nursing schools. There were only two such schools in Nova Scotia in 1914, at the Victoria General Hospital in Halifax and St. Joseph's Hospital in Glace Bay, but many Nova Scotian nurses trained in nursing schools elsewhere: in New Brunswick, Prince Edward Island, and Newfoundland but also in Montreal, Toronto, and the United States. Other Nova Scotian hospitals trained nurses but only in two-year programs, so their graduates had to complete a third year elsewhere to be recognized as what were later designated "registered" nurses.[26]

While Macdonald's requirements appeared to be strict, she did in fact make exceptions. Despite her requirement that nurses be unmarried, for example, she accepted at least five married Nova Scotian women for overseas service. Two of them clearly joined because they wanted to be near their husbands, who were physicians serving in RAMC hospitals in England. When Dr. Oscar Donovan transferred into the CAMC and was posted to No. 7 CSH in France, however, his wife, Lela (Hamm) Donovan, decided to go home. Similarly, when Dr. Charles Anderson returned home to Halifax, apparently for health reasons, his wife, Edith (Crockett) Anderson, understandably went with him.

The other three married nurses that Macdonald accepted had different situations. Annie MacDonald joined the CAMCNS in April 1916 despite being over age and having a husband and two children at home in Sydney Mines. Donalda Jean Campbell of Big Island, Pictou County, who had married Lawrence Campbell just before he enlisted in the CEF, joined the CAMCNS and went overseas but returned to Canada in December 1917, while he continued to serve with No. 3 Canadian Field Ambulance until returning home in April 1919. Edyth Andrews, a Liverpool nurse with eight months' CAMC experience, joined the CAMCNS in July 1918, leaving behind her husband, who had tried to enlist but was found to be physically unfit, and two children. She didn't go overseas, however, serving with the MD 6 Training Depot and CHH in Halifax until February 1919.

Macdonald did not accept male nurses, presumably reflecting the then-popular belief that nursing was a woman's profession, even though at least some nursing schools—including the one at Dalhousie University—had been training men since at least 1908. Male nurses could join the CEF but not the CAMCNS and served in hospitals and other medical units but only as stretcher bearers or hospital orderlies and were paid about half of what women were.[27] It is not known how many trained male nurses served in the war, but at least six of them were Nova Scotians: Adam Cruikshank, Arthur Leslie, Neil MacLean, Simon Mury, Charles Redmond and James Wall. One of them—Neil MacLean—was killed during the Battle of Courcelette in October 1916 and may be the only Canadian male nurse known to have been killed in the war. Simon Mury, who was from West Arichat, Richmond County, and likely trained at the VGH or St. Joseph's Hospital, was the only Acadian male nurse to serve overseas as an orderly in No. 7 CSH and No. 3 Canadian General Hospital (CGH). I also include a seventh man, Albert Drummond, who had moved with his family from Scotland to Halifax. When he enlisted in the CAMC in December 1916, he claimed to be a nurse, but he was not hospital-trained and later described himself as a masseur. Even so, he served in No. 3 and No. 14 Canadian Field Ambulance units in France and No. 15 Canadian Field Ambulance in England.

Similarly, Macdonald did not accept female doctors and when three of them—Margaret Parks, Evelyn Windsor and Margaret MacKenzie—applied to join the CAMCNS, Macdonald only accepted them because they had previously trained as nurses. This may seem odd, but the probable explanation is that the CAMCNS was, at its title indicates, a nursing service. The real question is why Carleton Jones did not accept female doctors in the CAMC as the RAMC had done, even though they were paid less than their male colleagues and ranked below RAMC subalterns, i.e., as lieutenants instead of captains.

Parks was an anaesthetist in Saint John, New Brunswick, and served in No. 1 CGH, which was commanded by Dr. Murray MacLaren, a prominent Saint John doctor. She also served in No. 2 CSH, No. 15 Ontario Military Hospital and No. 1 Canadian Casualty Clearing Station (CCCS) but only as a nurse. Windsor was from Montreal but was a physician in Calgary when she joined the CAMCNS in London in 1916 and quickly transferred into the RAMC.[28] MacKenzie was from Prince Edward Island and was a 1904 graduate of the VGH School of Nursing and a 1913 graduate of the medical school of St. Luke's Hospital in New York. She joined the QAIMNS in 1917 and served in RAMC No. 24 General Hospital in France and No. 48 Casualty Clearing Station. In February 1918 she transferred into the CAMCNS and served in England for a year until becoming seriously ill and returning home.[29]

Meanwhile, Macdonald had to cope with "certain civilian women" who, as Sir Andrew Macphail, a prominent physician, medical professor at McGill University and author of *Official History of the Canadian Forces in the Great War 1914–19: The Medical Service* (Ottawa, 1925), put it, "appeared...with no better credential than a verbal message or a personal telegram."[30] Most of them were rejected, but in 1916 Macdonald accepted nineteen women who weren't nurses at all but were designated "home sisters" because they provided valuable support services such as housekeeping for the nurses. They were entitled to the pay and allowances of nurses but not the rank. One of them was Roberta MacAdams, a trained dietician who served in No. 15 CSH in England until being elected to the Alberta legislature in 1917.[31]

Macdonald appears to have favoured Nova Scotian nurses, especially if they were from Pictou County. When the 118 nurses (plus Macdonald) went overseas with the first contingent in October 1914, only 9 were Nova Scotians and, perhaps not surprisingly, 4 of them—Margaret "Pearl" Fraser (New Glasgow), Harriet Graham (New Glasgow), Rosanna "Myrtle" Grattan (Pictou) and Janet Macdonald

(Big Island)—were from Pictou County. Janet Macdonald was also Margaret Macdonald's cousin and had grown up in Margaret's family home as a sister.

In the course of the war twelve Nova Scotian nurses, not including Margaret Macdonald, served as hospital matrons. Four of them (Pearl Fraser, Harriet Graham, Janet Macdonald and Elizabeth Ross) were from Pictou County, three (Jessie Jaggard, Katherine MacLatchy and Annie Strong) were from Kings County, two (Elizabeth Doyle and Laura Hubley) were from Halifax County, plus Louise Brock from Cape Breton County, Sarah MacIsaac from Antigonish, and Carolyn Viets from Digby. Perhaps not coincidentally, two of them (Jaggard and MacLatchy) were cousins of Sir Robert Borden, the prime minister, but all of these matrons were qualified and proved to be good choices.

Meanwhile, the Canadian Red Cross promptly established an overseas headquarters in London to establish new and support existing hospitals and convalescent homes. The most significant one was the Canadian Red Cross Hospital (DCRC) established by the Duchess of Connaught, whose husband was a son of Queen Victoria and served as the governor general of Canada from 1911 to 1916. It was built on the estate of Viscount Waldorf Astor, a wealthy American, and his wife, Lady Astor, at Taplow in Berkshire, near London. It was later enlarged and was redesignated No. 15 CGH. Most Canadian nurses were posted there for orientation before going on to serve in other hospitals.

Macdonald was, of course, well aware that the British Red Cross and the St. John Ambulance Association (SJAA) had joined in 1909 to form Voluntary Aid Detachments (VADs) to support nurses in the RAMC and that Canada's Department of Militia and Defence had authorized the SJAA in 1911 to do so as well.[32] The SJAA began "actively promoting voluntary aid nursing programs" in 1913, and when the war broke out, Canadian (and Newfoundland) VADs wanted to participate.[33] There wasn't much need of nursing support until the spring of 1915, however, when Canada's first division and the Newfoundland Regiment went into action in France and Gallipoli and wounded and ill soldiers began arriving home, requiring convalescent care. Some VADs subsequently travelled to London on their own and applied directly to the British VAD organization and were welcomed. Most women could not afford to do that, of course.

Historian Linda Quiney claims that Macdonald "refused to accept Canadian VADS" in the CAMC's overseas hospitals, fearing that they "could undermine the military discipline in the wards and the status" of trained nurses.[34] By September 1916, however, the number of casualties was so enormous that the first contingent of sixty Canadian VADs went overseas to serve in British military hospitals in England and France.[35] That reflected the fact that "the handful" of British VADs "who had gone to help on the Western Front had proved their worth" and "anyone who had had three months' hospital experience at home...would have the chance to go abroad."[36] Carleton Jones followed suit in April 1917, when he authorized the employment of fifteen VADs in Canadian overseas hospitals "for work in the recreation huts and as secretaries, and in Canadian-based hospitals."[37] According to Ethel McCarthy, another group was sent "for duty" in British units in February 1918.[38]

Macdonald did not object to VADs serving in military convalescent hospitals in Canada, however, because they were employed by the Military Hospitals Commission, created in 1915 to provide convalescent care to returning veterans, and were not included in the CAMCNS. The first VADs to serve in a Halifax military hospital, Pine Hill Convalescent Hospital, were Marion Doull, who had served in the QAIMNS in England, and Edith Pyke, both Nova Scotians, and Madeline Scott, who was English and a friend of Doull and Pyke.[39] When Halifax's hospitals were overwhelmed with patients injured in the Halifax explosion, Clara MacIntosh, the superintendent of the Nova Scotian branch of the VAD, was able to provide more than 191 women, some of whom were untrained college students.

That resulted in the Department of Militia and Defence's giving "formal recognition" of the VADs' "Military Service" in 1918, establishing the Women's Aid Detachment. By the end of the war approximately 2,000 Canadian VADs had served in Canada and about

500 Canadian and Newfoundland VADs had served in RAMC hospitals or in "assorted other roles," such as driving Red Cross ambulances in France, working in Red Cross recreation huts, or staffing the Red Cross rest home for nurses in Boulogne.[40]

As has already been noted, some Canadian nurses chose to travel to England and join the QAIMNS, the British army's nursing service. There is no accurate number of how many Canadian nurses did this, but Toman estimates that "at least" 313 Canadian and Newfoundland nurses did so.[41] The requirement was that they be British, meaning a citizen of one of the Commonwealth countries, between twenty-five and thirty-five years of age, have at least three years' training and service in a civil hospital having not fewer than one hundred beds, and be able to "satisfy the Nursing Board that as regards education and character and social status she is a fit person to enter the QAIMNS."[42]

Macdonald did not discourage this and in fact cooperated, appointing Jean Gunn, the supervisor of nurses at Toronto General Hospital, as the contact for nurses wishing to take that route. No doubt she calculated that at least some of them would eventually transfer to the CAMCNS because QAIMNS nurses weren't paid as well as Canadian nurses and did not have officer status. Among them were at least seven Nova Scotians: Frances Dodd (Bridgeport), Elva Gunn (Gore), Eunice Harrison (Southampton), Myrtle Howe (Nictaux), Marie Macdonell (Little Brook), Margaret McNeill (Aylesford) and Katherine White (Moser River).[43]

At least one Nova Scotian nurse—Carolyn Winnifred Viets[44]—appears to have joined Britain's Territorial Force Nursing Service (TFNS), a branch of the British Army's Territorial Force, a reserve unit that trained annually with the territorial army and was affiliated with the VAD. Women who joined the TFNS had to have completed at least three years of training in a recognized hospital, be twenty-three years of age or older, and be unmarried or widowed, with no dependants, although exceptions were made. During the war TFNS nurses worked alongside QAIMNS nurses in military medical units in Britain, France, Belgium, Malta, Gibraltar, Cairo, Salonika, Mesopotamia and East Africa.

At least seven qualified Nova Scotian nurses (Jessie Cann, Sara Corning, Lydia Ferguson, Minnie Hunt, Annie Killam, Evaline MacDonald and Helen Hastings Perry) served overseas in the American Red Cross or other non-governmental organizations. Elizabeth Belle Ross, also a trained nurse, joined the Société Française de Secours aux Blessés Militaires (SFSBM)—the French Red Cross—until transferring into the CAMCNS in London in February 1916. The SFSBM also accepted Katharine McLennan, who was neither a trained nurse nor a VAD but served in several hospitals in France and Germany. I include them all.

CHAPTER 1

Going Overseas

The first Canadian nurses to go overseas sailed from Quebec City with the first contingent of 30,617 troops[45] of the Canadian Expeditionary Force (CEF) on the afternoon of October 3, 1914. They had travelled from Valcartier the day before and were quartered overnight in the nearby Parc Savard Immigration Hospital.[46] Notwithstanding frequent claims that 100 nurses accompanied the soldiers, the Canadian Expeditionary Force Nursing Sisters Nominal Roll (October 4, 1914) clearly lists Margaret Macdonald and 119 nurses.[47] All of them were attached to No. 1 Canadian General Hospital (CGH), No. 2 CGH, or the Clearing Hospital—a unit from Liverpool, Nova Scotia, originally designated No. 2 Clearing Hospital—but they did not all travel together.

Macdonald and some of the nurses of No. 2 CGH sailed on the *Franconia*, the flagship of the convoy, and the *Virginian,* while others from No. 1 CGH sailed on the *Scandinavian.* The forty-five nurses of No. 1 Canadian Stationary Hospital (CSH) and No. 2 CSH, who had been drawn from No. 1 CGH and No. 2 CGH, sailed on the *Athena*, the *Grampian*, and the *Scotian.* The Clearing Hospital sailed on the *Megantic* with eleven officers and seventy-five other ranks but the anticipated ten to twelve nurses were not listed in its nominal roll until it was designated No. 1 Canadian Casual Clearing Station (CCCS) in England prior to going to France in February 1915.[48]

Nurse Mabel Clint, attached to No. 1 CGH, later recalled that, when they sailed from Quebec on October 2, "it was a beautiful

Canadian autumn day, the surrounding hills and woods forming a background of brilliant colour, a warm purple haze hanging over the ships."[49] When the 540 volunteers of the Newfoundland Regiment arrived on the *Florizel* on October 6, the fleet of thirty-three troopships, protected by ten Royal Navy warships, set sail for England. Although many inevitably suffered from seasickness, it must have been an exciting experience. Dr. Robert Manion, a physician from Fort William, Ontario, who went overseas with the 21st Battalion a year later, might well have been speaking for the first contingent when he recalled that "we were not long away from land till a fairly heavy swell made some of the uninitiated sea voyagers feel all the pangs of that nauseating illness, mal de mere, and one of the nurses sitting in a deck chair, looking away off over the swelling billows, said languidly: 'If the Germans torpedoed us now, I wouldn't even put on a life preserver.'"[50]

Most adjusted after a couple of days, but the *Franconia* was crowded, and at least one officer, Lieutenant Colonel George Nasmith, complained that the nurses spoiled what could have been an enjoyable journey:

> There seemed to be about a thousand aboard the *Franconia*—the real number was about a hundred, but they multiplied by their ubiquity; they swarmed everywhere; sometimes they filled the lounge so that the poor Major or Colonel could not get in for his afternoon cup of tea. The daily lectures for officers, particularly on subjects like "the Geneva Convention" and "Hygiene" which they might have found useful held little attraction for them.[51]

According to Mabel Clint, however, they did in fact attend lectures on "war nursing, sanitation of camps, and military routines."[52]

What really annoyed Nasmith was the perversity of the nurses when given the rank of an officer and being freed from all hospital restraint. "At the concerts few officers could obtain seats," he claimed, "and a few of us were mean enough to wish that it would get rough enough to put some of the nurses temporarily down and out." In his opinion the nurses were in a doubly fortunate position in that they could demand the rights of both officers and women, what happened to be advantageous.[53] Accordingly, when the officers on the *Franconia* decided to organize a dinner party on the last evening at sea "before the gallant ship's company was scattered, few to meet again or return to Canada,"[54] their first plan was not to include the nurses. "Other counsels" prevailed, however, and it was proposed to invite "a limited number" until they realized that "this would have caused all sorts of petty jealousies and heart burnings." A compromise "was effected by asking them all" and the dinner was "a great success."[55]

Lieutenant Colonel Robert Rudolf, a prominent Nova Scotian physician who also went overseas with the first contingent, took a more tolerant attitude towards the enthusiasm of the nurses, acknowledging that they had "mixed things up a bit at first" but only because applying military discipline "as usually applied to officers of that rank was a misfit."[56] And to be fair, Nasmith later acknowledged that "in their daily routine, after the strain of heavy engagements and even after being subjected to bombing," the nurses "played the game and played it well," and Rudolf conceded that the nurses had "soon settled into the usual routine of military hospital work."[57]

Upon arrival at Plymouth, the nurses travelled to London, where they were housed at St. Thomas' Hospital, where Florence Nightingale had founded her training school for nurses in 1850. They also became acquainted with British military nursing at Millbank hospital and the fact that the CAMCNS came under the "overall nursing authority" of the QAIMNS. That meant that Matron-in-Chief Macdonald answered to its Matron-in-Chief, Maud McCarthy. Meanwhile, they quickly found themselves "caught up in a whirlwind of sightseeing, theatre parties, receptions, and teas."[58]

By October 1914 the war had been raging for more than three months, and the RAMC had learned that there was a need for hospitals other than the general hospitals that were large, situated well behind the front lines, and required between seventy and one hundred nurses. The result was the creation of stationary hospitals, which were smaller, closer to the front lines, could be moved if necessary, and only required a matron and sixteen nurses, although Adami claims that the two first stationary hospitals—Nos. 1 and 2 CSH—drew forty-five nurses from No. 1 CGH and No. 2 CGH before going to France.[59] Smaller still were casualty clearing stations, small facilities that treated emergency cases close to the front lines but were accessible to ambulances or close to railway lines so that they could evacuate wounded soldiers to hospitals farther behind the lines or to England for more extensive medical aid.[60] They began with fewer than a dozen nurses, growing to as many as forty nurses by 1917.[61]

The first Canadian hospital to go to France was No. 2 CSH in November 1914, followed by No. 1 CSH and No. 1 CCCS in February 1915, No. 2 CGH in March 1915, No. 1 CGH in May 1915, and No. 3 CGH in June 1915. By 1918 these six Canadian hospitals had expanded to thirty: sixteen general hospitals, ten stationary hospitals and four casualty clearing stations. There were also five hospital ships on which military nurses served, returning convalescent soldiers to

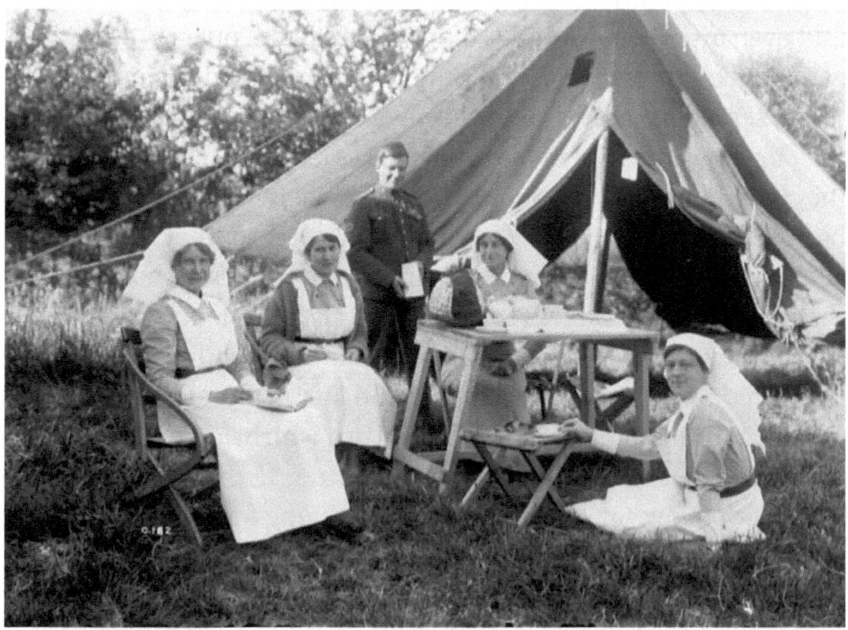

Nurses, No. 3 Casualty Clearing Station, July, 1916. [CANADA, DEPT. OF NATIONAL DEFENCE/LIBRARY AND ARCHIVES CANADA]

Canada,[62] and as the war dragged on, growing numbers of nurses served in convalescent military and public and private hospitals in England and Canada.

No. 2 CSH was posted to Le Touquet, a resort on the English Channel in November 1914, months before any Canadian troops went to France.[63] Ethel Ridley, Macdonald's assistant at Valcartier, was appointed matron, presumably because Macdonald wanted an experienced military nurse in charge of the first hospital unit to go to France.[64] Ridley led the first twenty of No. 2's nurses, but they were followed four days later by the other fifteen nurses, three of whom (Pearl Fraser, Harriet Graham and Myrtle Grattan) were Nova Scotians from Pictou County. Ten more nurses were posted to the hospital in March 1915, but within a year they were transferred to England.

Graham reported in December 1914 that "we have the most beautiful hospital you could imagine, and we are simply proud of ourselves, for [being] the FIRST Canadian Hospital to be in France." They had been "awfully busy" reorganizing the hotel as a hospital and cleaning it, but "we all love it." Lieutenant Colonel Adam Shillington, its commanding officer, had decided that each ward should be named after a province, and Nova Scotia got "the prettiest ward, with seventy-five beds and the most important place. We all were extremely pleased."[65] Graham also reported that "we have a dandy crowd of girls and a very nice crowd of officers, and our men are as willing as can be, though most of them are untrained."[66]

The men to whom she was referring are seldom mentioned because they were non-commissioned soldiers. Some of them were medical students, and a few were actually trained male nurses who were only allowed to work as orderlies, assisting the nurses by making beds, moving patients, assisting in operating rooms and working at night so that the nurses could rest, especially in crisis situations. By November 12, 1918, 12,243 "other ranks" were serving in the CAMC.[67]

Although it was very early innings in the war, Fraser and Graham were already getting a sense of what it was going to be like because the first battle of Ypres was taking place. According to Mabel Clint, who had been transferred into No. 2 CSH, it and the other hospitals at Boulogne received 20,000 casualties in one week.[68] Ambulances usually arrived at night, so that was the busiest time, even though Graham had been on duty all day. She was writing a letter at ten o'clock just before they arrived:

> ...but I see where we don't get to bed tonight. By the time we get the poor souls into bed and half way clean, and a dressing done, it's [*sic*] morning before you know it, and the poor creatures...are so filthy, and many times just alive with vermin. Pearl said tonight: "Isn't it funny, in our hospitals we despised men who were dirty, and here the worse they are, the better we like them." When they say, "keep away sister, I'm so dirty, but I have been in the trenches and I haven't had a bath for so many weeks," I just feel like saying, "I honor your dirt."[69]

Continuing her letter the next day, Graham described a conversation with one soldier, who was

> just a lad of eighteen, and the nicest kind of a kid. He told me his two pals were shot and killed. I said, "weren't you awfully afraid?" "Yes, sister," he said, "I was awfully afraid at first...but I soon got over it." ...He then asked me if it would be long before he could go back. "Why," I said, "do you want to go back?" He just looked at me and said: "Does anybody want to go to Hell, sister?" And, poor kid, he will have to go back because he is not very badly injured.[70]

The nurses quickly discovered that convalescing soldiers needed more than medical care, however, and began purchasing comforts and treats for them. Graham reported that "I spend all the spare pennies I can find on cigarettes for them, poor boys, it seems to do more to quiet their nerves than anything else." That wasn't enough, however, so she appealed to the New Glasgow Red Cross Society, explaining that "although our Hospital is very well equipped for active service, any additional hospital supplies are always welcome."[71]

According to Adruenna "Addie" Tupper, a nurse from Bridgewater who was also serving at No. 2 CSH, which had moved to Outreau in April 1915,

> every sister of us spends every franc she has for the things they need: cigarettes, tooth-wash and brushes, treats of cake etc, books and papers. Oh, the need of money! My tent-mate has an uncle who supplies her with great boxes of cigarettes, biscuits, toilet powder, and anything she suggests, also sends her good big cheques. Miss [Annie] Strong had 16 shillings sent her yesterday and bought combs, brushes and toothbrushes with it. These things are as necessary as socks.[72]

When Tupper's health began to fail a few months later, she was sent home on leave in November 1915 on a hospital ship with other nurses caring for eight hundred convalescent soldiers. Tupper returned overseas and was serving in England when she was awarded the Royal Red Cross 1st Class but fell ill with pneumonia and died in December 1916.[73]

Other nurses appealed to other societies for help as well, with the result that local women's groups collected hospital supplies such as sheets, hospital shirts, hot water bottle covers, socks, mittens, bandages, handkerchiefs, nightingales (simple garments, often knitted, crocheted or flannel), housewives (sewing kits) and other necessaries. Harry Hiltz, a lieutenant in the 25th Battalion, wrote to the Red Cross Society at home in Kingsport, Nova Scotia, in February 1916 to report that "the various hospital staffs around here speak very highly of the help you people give them in making many comforts for the wounded," adding that when the British hospitals recently ran short of materials, especially clothing, the Canadian hospitals were able to supply them.[74]

Meanwhile, the brothers of Pearl Fraser and Harriet Graham had also gone to England with the first contingent in October 1914, and remarkably, they managed to get together with their sisters for Christmas. Given a few days' leave, Alistair Fraser and Wendell Graham crossed over to Boulogne, where their sisters had "borrowed" an ambulance from Le Touquet and were joined by Charles Sutherland, another Pictou County friend, who was in England representing the Nova Scotia Steel and Coal Company. A couple of days after their Christmas dinner, the boys were driven back to Boulogne in the ambulance and returned to England. As Pictou County historian James Cameron says, "the incident had no military significance—but as a circumvention of military security and red tape it was a unique accomplishment."[75] No. 1 CSH moved to Wimereux on the outskirts of Boulogne in March 1915 but only briefly, before being transferred in August 1915 to the island of Lemnos, the British army's logistical and medical base during the Gallipoli campaign, and Salonika in March 1916. Its experience there will be discussed later.

The third Canadian medical unit to go to France was No. 1 CCCS, which took possession of Fort Gassion, a former prison at Aire-sur-la-Lys, near Saint-Omer, the headquarters of the British First Army. It was commanded by Colonel F. S. L. Ford, a physician from Milton, Nova Scotia, who had nine years' experience in CAMC. Its personnel consisted of eleven officers (including Ford), six nurses and seventy-five other ranks. One of its nurses was Minnie Asenath Follette of Ward's Brook, Cumberland County, a 1909 graduate of the VGH School of Nursing, who had CAMC experience when she joined the CAMCNS in September 1914. When Joseph Hayes, a prominent Nova Scotian doctor who served with the 85th Battalion—a Nova Scotian infantry battalion—visited Fort Gassion in March 1915, it was "filthy and in a dilapidated condition,"[76] but within two days its personnel had cleaned the building and unpacked its equipment in time to receive 550 casualties from the heavy fighting in the First Battle of Ypres. The unit performed so well that Ford was awarded the CMG (Order of St. Michael and St. George), the first to be awarded to a Canadian in the field.

No. 3 CGH, organized by McGill University's medical school, the oldest and most prestigious in Canada, went overseas in May 1915 with members of its medical faculty and seventy-two nurses chosen equally from the Royal Victoria Hospital and the Montreal General Hospital.[77] Their matron was Katherine MacLatchy of Grand Pré,

Nova Scotia, who was a cousin of Sir Robert Borden. No. 3 CGH was established at Camiers,[78] one of the villages close to Étaples where No. 1 CGH and several British hospitals were established. It arrived just in time in August to receive its first patients: 2,000 casualties from the Second Battle of Ypres in June. That was followed in late September by the admission of "more than 1,000 patients" from the Battle of Loos.

No. 3 CGH was a tent hospital, and when in October a fierce storm of "rain and wind swept the tents...tearing the canvas, pulling pegs from the soft ground, and flooding many of the wards" so badly that "everything was floating," the nurses had to carry out their work in "mud almost to the knees."[79] The result was that thirty nurses were temporarily transferred to hospitals in England while wooden huts were built and they "moved from their sodden tents without regret."[80]

On the evening of December 24, 1915, No. 3's first Christmas Eve in France, carollers from the RAMC No. 18 General Hospital, "with mandolin and banjo accompanists, made their way to the grounds of the McGill unit and invited the Canadians to join in welcoming Christmas Day." Describing the occasion, an unnamed diarist wrote: "It was a sight not to be forgotten. Officers and nursing sisters stood in the deep mud to sing 'God Save the King,' then, forming inner and outer circles, all joined in singing 'Auld Lang Syne.'" Next morning divine service was held in the hospital's operating room, which had been stripped of all that pertained to surgery and decorated with holly, ivy, pine branches, and mistletoe. Later, the officers and nurses dined together, all regretting the absence of many who had sailed with the unit from Montreal, now on duty elsewhere. Similarly, in the sergeants' and men's messes, where special dinners were served, those who had received commissions or returned to Canada were sorely missed.[81]

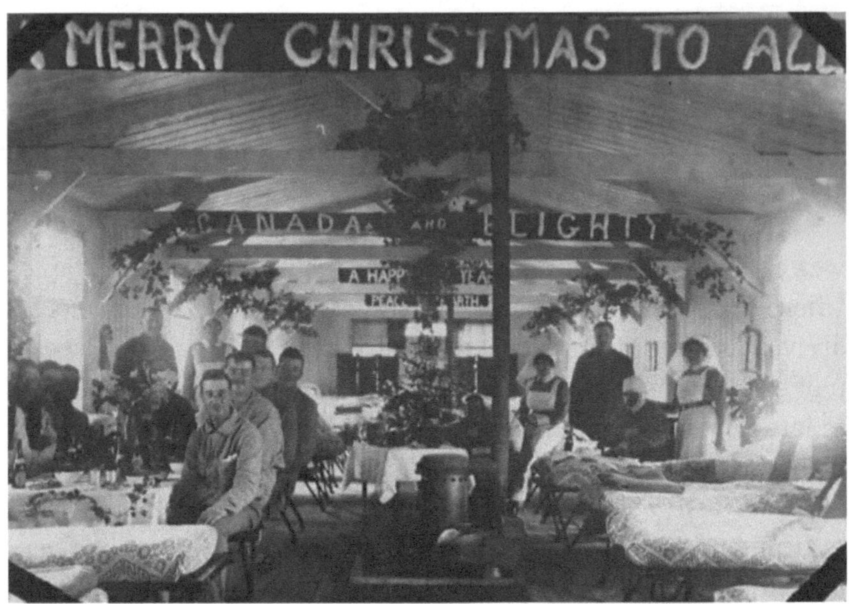

Unidentified nursing sisters with patients in a Christmas-decorated ward, No. 2 Canadian General Hospital, Le Tréport, France. [ÉDITIONS ARNAULT/ALICE ISAACSON FONDS/LIBRARY AND ARCHIVES CANADA/E007150692]

No. 3's Christmas gift, albeit belated, was that it was moved in January 1916 to a Jesuit college on the outskirts of Boulogne, replacing the RAMC No. 22 General Hospital. While extensive renovations were being made, thirty of the nurses were transferred temporarily to hospitals in England.[82] They returned just in time for the infamous Battle of the Somme that began on July 1 and resulted in massive British casualties, seven thousand of whom were treated by No. 3 CGH. It also treated some two thousand patients when the Canadian Corps successfully captured Vimy Ridge in April 1917.[83] Months later, in the "cold, moonlit night" of December 22, 1917, German aircraft attacked Boulogne. No bombs hit the hospital, although four "crashed" into nearby huts occupied by the Canadian Army Service Corps, killing forty men and wounding several others.[84]

On a happier note, on Christmas Day 1915 "special dinners were served to the 1,300 patients in their respective wards," after which the nurses served dinner to the other ranks in the Canadian Red Cross hut, then the officers and nurses dined together in the recreation hut which had been "polished, cleaned and decorated" with "holly, mistletoe, evergreens, and ivy...and someone had secured gorgeous roses for the table." Afterward the tables were moved, and the hospital orchestra played dance music until 11:45 P.M. The next day, the convalescent patients celebrated Boxing Day in the Red Cross hut, and on the afternoon of December 30 MacLatchy and her nurses were "at home" to a number of guests. Among them were Georgina Pope, Macdonald's predecessor as matron-in-chief, who had transferred into the CAMCNS and had been matron of No. 2 CSH since December 1917; the matron of the No. 5 American Base Hospital, and "many" other officers serving in medical units in the area.[85]

By the end of the war, No. 3 CGH had admitted 81,689 medical patients and 52,389 wounded and had carried out 11,395 operations with a death rate of less than 1 percent.[86] When Sir William Peterson, the president of McGill University, visited it in August 1916 he was told by British authorities that No. 3 was "the best medical unit in France."[87] That was probably true, although Andrew Beckett and Edward J. Harvey, writing many years later, more modestly claimed only that it was known as "one of the best medical units within the armies in France."[88] The British were no doubt influenced by their awareness that McGill's most distinguished alumnus was Sir William Osler, the regius professor of medicine at Oxford University, who had been one of the founders of the Johns Hopkins Hospital and medical school in Baltimore and is still regarded as the "Father of Modern Medicine."[89] Among No. 3's physicians were Dr. Francis Scrimger, the only Canadian medical officer to receive the Victoria Cross for his "greatest devotion to duty among the wounded at the front" during the "very heavy fighting" at Vimy Ridge,[90] and Dr. John McCrae, a highly respected surgeon who became better known for writing "In Flanders Fields."

The University of Toronto's medical school, the second best in Canada, was organized in March 1915 as No. 4 Canadian General Hospital and went to England with No. 3 CGH in May 1915. After five months at the Shorncliffe Military Hospital, it was posted to Salonika in Greece and is discussed later. Three smaller universities—Queen's, Laval, and Dalhousie—organized stationary hospitals in September 1915, but Laval was upgraded to become No. 6 CGH in December 1915, and Queen's was upgraded to become No. 7 CGH in January 1916.

No. 7 CSH (Dalhousie) was the largest and most important university hospital unit in the Maritime provinces. Its commanding officer was Dr. John Stewart, a prominent Halifax physician and professor of surgery at Dalhousie despite being sixty-seven years of age.[91] Most of No. 7's doctors and nurses and its dentist were from the VGH Medical School. Laura Hubley of St. Margarets Bay, an 1898 graduate of the VGH School of Nursing who had already joined the CAMCNS, nursed at the CMH and was matron of CHH in Halifax, was appointed matron of No. 7 CSH. All twenty-seven of its nurses—chosen from the eighty who applied[92]—were Nova Scotians and graduates of the VGH School of Nursing or St. Joseph's Hospital in Glace Bay. A Catholic hospital, St. Joseph's was the second largest in Nova Scotia and the only one other than the VGH that had a three-year nursing training school.[93] Almost all of the 121 other ranks in No. 7 were also Nova Scotians.[94]

While undergoing initial training in Halifax, No. 7 was billeted in the old Medical College building on the corner of Robie and College Streets, with its mess in the Maritime Business College next door. When it departed Halifax on December 31, 1915, to go overseas, a large crowd from all over the province gathered at the North Street train station to see them off, joined by the Halifax garrison's regimental bands and the pipes of the 63rd militia regiment. "The departure at one time of so many professional men and women, who stood high in the confidence of the people of Halifax and Nova Scotia was," as Joseph Hayes observed, "a poignant reminder of the serious proportions assumed by the Great War."[95]

Upon arrival in England, No. 7 CSH was initially stationed at the Shorncliffe Military Hospital before moving in June 1916 to Le Havre in France, then Harfleur until May 1917, Arques until April 1918, Étaples very briefly to May 1918, Rouen until September 1918, and finally Camiers to February 1919. While at Arques, its 379 patients included 13 German officers. The nurse in charge of them was Wilhelmina "Irene" Thompson from Glencoe, Pictou County, who kept a diary.[96] She described the unexpected visit on July 3, 1917, of King George V, the Prince of Wales and Sir William Robertson, the chief of the Imperial General Staff, who were driving to the British army's nearby headquarters when the king recognized the Nova Scotia flag on a building and stopped because he had spent some time as a midshipman in Halifax and remembered the kind hospitality he had received. He and his party remained to help celebrate Stewart's birthday and to speak to the staff and patients, and when they left, the hospital's piper appeared in kilt and full regalia and played "Will Ye No Come Back Again."[97]

St. Francis Xavier University, a small Catholic university in Antigonish, also offered a hospital unit in March 1916 despite not having either a medical school or a school of nursing. In fact, its total enrolment in the 1914–15 academic year had only been 181 students, which

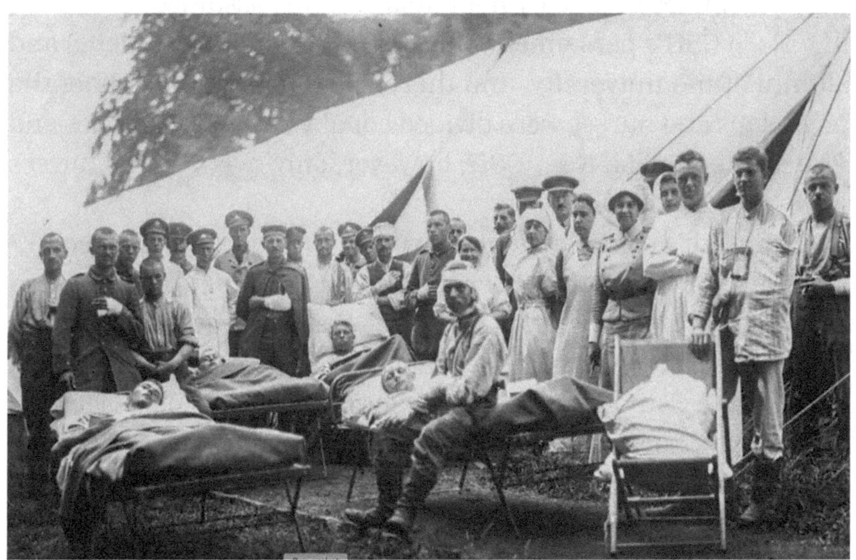

German wounded with Dalhousie medical and nursing staff. June 1917, Arques, France. [DALHOUSIE ARCHIVES]

had fallen to 97 after almost half of its male students had joined the army. Even so, Rev. Hugh MacPherson, St. FX's president, thought it should do something because he considered the school to be the major English-speaking Catholic university in the country. The idea of a hospital originated, however, with Dr. John Stuart Carruthers, the medical officer at the marine hospital in Pubnico, Nova Scotia, whose father-in-law, Senator Adam Brown Crosby, a prominent Catholic, was a Halifax businessman, a Conservative member of parliament from 1908 to 1911 and a friend of Sir Robert Borden, who appointed him to the Senate in January 1917.[98]

According to James Cameron, the university's historian, MacPherson's vice president, Rev. J. J. Tompkins, also "rejoiced that the government would pay all expenses while St. FX got 'all the glory' from...the Atlantic to the Pacific" while others believed that a Catholic hospital unit would also protect young Catholic men who served in it from "grave moral as well as physical dangers" to which they would be exposed if they served in combat battalions.[99] There appears not to have been any concern about such dangers to the twenty-six nurses, at least not initially. It was assumed, of course, that No. 9 CSH's personnel would be predominantly students and alumni of the university, and therefore Catholic, but in fact the physicians and nurses were divided equally between Catholics and Protestants. Unlike No. 7 CSH, however, only twenty of its nurses were Nova Scotians.[100]

The unit's commanding officer was Dr. Roderick MacLeod,[101] a native of Dunvegan in Inverness County, a graduate of St. FX and the University of New York's medical school. He was only a general practitioner, however, albeit in Halifax, with no militia experience, but he was a Catholic. The matron, Sarah Catherine MacIsaac, was well chosen, however. A graduate of Mount Saint Bernard College in Antigonish and St. Joseph's Hospital School of Nursing, she had overseen nursing services for St. Joseph's operating room for three years before completing post-graduate training at Mercy Hospital in Chicago and was assistant matron at Mount Zion Hospital in San Francisco when she returned home to join No. 9.[102]

No. 9's medical officers and nurses were sent to Halifax in May 1916 to enable the physicians to participate in a CAMC training course while its nurses were posted briefly to local hospitals before they departed for England in June 1916. As James Cameron acknowledges, No. 9's overseas experience proved to be "not entirely satisfactory."[103] Upon its arrival, it was attached to the Duchess of Connaught Red Cross Hospital (later redesignated No. 12 CGH) at the CEF's Bramshott Camp in Hampshire until October 1917, when military authorities ordered that it merge with No. 12 CGH. When St. FX officials protested, No. 9 was sent in December 1917 to Longuenesse, near Saint-Omer, in France.[104]

It got off to a shocking start when MacLeod contracted spinal meningitis from a cut and died on January 5. He was succeeded by his second-in-command, Dr. Henry Kendall, a physician in Sydney who was a Protestant and an alumnus of Mount Allison University, a Methodist institution, and had no connection with St. FX. His daughter, Helen Kendall, had graduated from Montreal's RVH School of Nursing in 1916, joined the CAMCNS, and served overseas in other hospitals in England and France. Dr. Kendall had strong political connections, however, having married a daughter of J. S. McLennan, a Montreal industrialist who had moved to Sydney, owned the *Sydney Daily Post* newspaper, and was an influential Conservative whom Sir Robert Borden had appointed to the Senate.[105]

In April 1918 No. 9 was moved to Étaples and was designated a "special" convalescent hospital, meaning that it would treat venereal disease. Venereal disease was an inevitable problem in all armies, but the CEF had the highest rate among the Allied troops.[106] Putting this in context, the number of Canadian soldiers infected with venereal disease during the war was virtually the same as the number who died in the war. What must have been especially embarrassing, at least to St. FX, was that the highest rate of infection in the CEF was in the 5th Brigade, whose four battalions—the 22nd and 24th (Montreal), the 25th (Nova Scotia) and the 26th (New Brunswick)—were predominantly Catholic.[107] St. FX's historian acknowledges that the unit was "really too ambitious for such a small college" because it lacked a medical school and "had little more than a tenuous connection to the college." What was worse, being assigned to a venereal disease hospital "was probably distasteful to a unit associated with a Catholic college"[108] and nurses were not allowed to serve in those hospitals.

Kendall's response was to arrange a transfer to No. 12 CGH. He was succeeded by Dr. Ronald St. John Macdonald, a St. FX alumnus who had joined No. 3 CGH in April 1915 and, perhaps not coincidentally, was the brother of Matron-in-Chief Margaret Macdonald. In September 1918 he was ordered to move No. 9 from Étaples to Camiers, but it received no patients until early February 1919 when it replaced No. 7 CSH, the Dalhousie hospital unit, which had also been functioning as a venereal disease hospital at Étaples, Rouen, and Camiers since April 1918.

One cannot help wondering, given that the rate of infection in the CEF was highest among Canadian soldiers from the Maritime provinces, if it was just coincidental that the three Canadian venereal disease hospitals were commanded by Nova Scotians. Indeed, the largest Canadian VD hospital was No. 3 CGH at Etchinghill, Kent, which had 1,060 beds. It was commanded from August 1916 to June 1919 by Lieutenant Colonel W. T. M. MacKinnon, a physician from Amherst, Nova Scotia, who became an authority on the subject.[109]

The impact on Nova Scotian and other nurses was that they were transferred to other hospitals because the CAMC thought it inappropriate for women to nurse men with venereal diseases. They were replaced by male orderlies but, according to historian Lyndsay Rosenthal, male orderlies "did not always provide the same level of care," and there was a shortage of them, with the result that patients were put to work under their direction.[110] No. 9 CSH and No. 7 CSH returned home in July 1919.

CHAPTER 2

Far from the Western Front

Meanwhile, three Canadian hospital units—No. 1 CSH, No. 3 CSH, and No. 5 CSH (later redesignated No. 7 CGH)—had been sent to the eastern Mediterranean in August 1915 to help cope with the heavy losses being incurred by the Anglo-French attempt to capture Gallipoli on the Ottoman Empire's strategic Dardanelles waterway. The decision to send Canadian hospitals to a region where there were no Canadian troops proved to be very controversial, although nearly 1,100 soldiers from the Newfoundland Regiment served there. Guy Carleton Jones, the CEF's director of medical services, recognized that CAMC resources should be kept in Britain and France but had yielded to the desperate appeal of Lieutenant General Sir Alfred Keogh, the RAMC's director general, given the dreadful situation in the Mediterranean at the time.

Sam Hughes, Minister of Militia and Defence, vigorously objected, however, arguing that Canadian medical resources should be used to support Canadian troops rather than be "at the disposal of the War Office," which constituted "subservience to Britain."[111] Nurse Mabel Clint, who had been transferred to No. 1 CSH, agreed with him, claiming in her postwar memoirs that "the majority" of the nurses concurred, fearing that they would "lose our identity and be side-tracked" if they were sent where there were no Canadian troops.[112]

Hughes commissioned Dr. Herbert Bruce, a prominent Toronto physician and a Conservative who had founded the Wellesley Hospital but had no military experience, to investigate the management of the CAMC. Not surprisingly, Bruce produced a highly critical report on its efficiency and its "subservience" to the War Office, so Hughes fired Jones and replaced him with Bruce. That was the last straw for Borden, who had had enough of Hughes by now and fired him, replacing him with Sir George Perley, one of Borden's closest and most reliable advisors.

The three units proceeded on the hospital ship *Asturias* to Malta in the Mediterranean anyway, where they arrived on August 8 only "to find that no instructions had been received there concerning their future movements." As Adami rightly observed, "everything associated with the brave but ill-fated Gallipoli expedition had in it an element of unpreparedness," which was "as true of the medical as of the military arrangements."[113]

They were then sent to Alexandria, in Egypt, where, "after a day of contradictory orders," No. 1 and No. 3 proceeded to Lemnos, a barren island in the eastern Mediterranean whose only merit was that it was the British army's logistical and medical base and was relatively close to Gallipoli, a vital Turkish position that the British, Australian, New Zealand and Newfoundland troops were trying to conquer. As historian Christine Hallett has put it, Lemnos was "not only a hostile and inhospitable environment; its administration as a military base exhibited all of the worst features of the badly-handled Gallipoli campaign."[114]

While the doctors of No. 1 and No. 3 sailed on "a transport," the seventy nurses—including their matrons, Eleanor Charleson and Jessie Jaggard—despite being officers, travelled on the *Delta*, a hospital ship that "had been used as a horse transport and had not since been cleaned."[115] Upon arrival, they established tent hospitals on a coastal plain that, according to Adami, "had been only recently vacated by a camp of some thousands of Egyptian labourers, not possessed of the most elementary ideas of camp sanitation. Nor... had any sanitary provisions been taken," and within eight days there were more than five hundred men in the hospital.[116]

Nor had any arrangements been made to provide the hospitals with food. According to Charleson, there was "nothing to eat except malted milk tablets" for two days until the navy arrived with food and water. That didn't last long, however, and No. 1's food consisted mainly of stew, pale gray bread, margarine instead of butter, canned milk and coffee, and the nurses "wrote consistently about how hungry they were."[117] Dysentery was rampant and, according to Clint, deaths became so numerous by October that a burial party stayed at the cemetery all day, fifty graves were being dug every night, and at one point "only three out of thirty-five nurses were on duty."[118]

Having said that, however, Clint reports that there was "an energetic and capable" home sister among No. 1's nurses who, "by dint of driving round the Island, discovering what could be obtained, visiting the liners in harbour, and...sending orders to Egypt and Malta to be delivered by next transport." By October sufficient and palatable meals were being provided, and "on Christmas night we sat down to as good and festive a dinner as our respective home hospitals could have served in Canada. It was the one and only British Christmas celebrated on Lemnos."[119]

No. 3 was another story. It was "widely acknowledged to be the least sanitary of the Canadian hospitals in the East, and likely of all Canadian hospitals throughout the war."[120] According to Kate Wilson, one of its nurses, conditions were appalling because of intense heat, a severe shortage of water that limited nurses to one quart (slightly more than a litre) every twenty-four hours for drinking and cleaning, and at night the nurses slept on army cots—as did the patients—under netting to ward off the "clouds of flies."[121] By September dysentery was "prevalent among the Officers, Nursing Sisters and personnel," with the result that "the strain on those members of the personnel who were still unaffected was very heavy."[122] Thirty-two of its nurses fell ill, and two died while twelve others had to be invalided to England.

The two who died were Mary Munro and Jessie Jaggard, No. 3's matron. When Munro died on September 7, 1915, she had the dubious distinction of being the first Canadian military nurse to die in the war. Jaggard died eighteen days later. Both were buried in the Portianou Military Cemetery. Jaggard was "much loved," according to Kate Wilson, because "with little thought for herself and a keen interest in her nursing staff," she "would go from hut to hut of her sleeping nurses, assuring herself that they were alright and not suffering from want of blankets when the nights were extra cold," and "forever she will remain in the hearts of those who were privileged to serve under her."[123] More than a hundred years later, in April 2018, Nova Scotia's House of Assembly unanimously adopted a resolution "honouring the devotion and courage" that Jaggard had "displayed during the Great War."[124]

Why was No. 3 CSH stricken more seriously than the other hospital units on Lemnos? Aside from "the lack of sanitary precautions taken and an unhealthy location,"[125] its commanding officer, Lieutenant Colonel Henry Casgrain, was a small-town physician whose only military medical experience was in the 1885 Northwest Rebellion. Worse, after No. 3 went to England in April 1915, it had no experience beyond the four months at Shorncliffe when it was sent to Lemnos. By comparison, No. 1 CSH had had some six months' experience in France before being sent to Lemnos. Within weeks Casgrain sent an urgent cable to London describing the situation, and the RAMC transferred No. 3 to Alexandria in February 1916, then to England in April 1916, and finally to France. And yet Clint claimed that she "never heard one [nurse] say that she was sorry to have served on Lemnos. That was real 'active service,' they said. We were very badly needed there."[126]

When Vera Brittain, the British poet who was serving as a VAD on HMHS *Britannic*, visited Lemnos in 1916 and saw the graves of Mary Munro and Jessie Jaggard, she was moved to write a poem "The Sisters' Graves at Lemnos," published in the *Oxford Magazine* (May 11, 1917) and in her collection, *Poems of the War and After* (London: Macmillan, 1934).

The Sisters' Graves At Lemnos[127]

("Fidelis ad extremum.")

O Golden Isle set in the deep-blue Ocean
With purple shadows flitting o'er thy crest,
I kneel to thee in reverent devotion
Of some who on thy bosom lie at rest!

Seldom they enter into song or story—
Poets praise the soldiers' might and deeds of war,
But few recall the Sisters, and the glory
Of women dead beneath a distant star.

No armies threatened in that lonely station,
They fought not fire or sword, or ruthless foe,
But heat and hunger, sickness and privation,
And Winter's deathly chill and blinding snow.

Till mortal frailty could endure no longer
Disease's ravages and climate's power,
In body weak but spirit ever stronger,
Courageously they stayed to meet their hour.

No blazing tribute through the wide world flying,
No rich reward of sacrifice they craved;
The only meed of their victorious dying
Lives in the hearts of humble men they saved;

Who, when in light the Final Dawn is breaking,
Still faithful, though the world's regard shall cease,
Will honour, splendid in triumphant waking,
The souls of women, lonely here at peace.

O Golden Isle with purple shadows falling
Across thy rocky shore and sapphire sea,
I shall not think of these without recalling
The Sisters sleeping on the heart of thee!

In November 1915 the British government sensibly began withdrawing its troops from Gallipoli and sent them to Salonika, a port and the major city in Macedonia in northwestern Greece, to deter Bulgaria from joining Germany and Austria-Hungary in an attack on nearby Serbia. Canada contributed three hospital units: No. 1 CSH, No. 4 CGH and No. 5 CGH. Rather oddly, No. 4 CGH and No. 5 CGH were the first to be sent despite neither of them having any experience outside of England, while No. 1 CSH, which had six months' experience in France and eight months at Lemnos, was the last to be transferred. Fortunately, No. 4 had been organized by the University of Toronto's Medical School and had administered the Shorncliffe Military Hospital in England. Also fortunately, its pathologist, Dr. J. J. Mackenzie, wrote frequent letters home to his wife describing his experiences, which she published in 1933.[128]

No. 4 sailed on the *Kildonan Castle*, a hospital ship that was first diverted to Suvla Bay at Gallipoli to pick up 670 British casualties and deliver them to Lemnos. According to an anonymous nurse who was there, that took longer than it should have because there were "not infrequent stops" en route to bury soldiers who died at sea. After disembarking the most seriously wounded patients in Malta, the ship returned to Suvla Bay and picked up more casualties before proceeding to Salonika.[129] According to Mackenzie, the RAMC authorities in Malta treated the nurses very badly, giving them hardly enough to eat, making them sleep in the same quarters as the servants, and making "very nasty remarks about them wearing a uniform with lieutenant's stars and receiving lieutenant's pay."[130]

When No. 4 reached Salonika in November, it was without seventeen of its nurses, who continued to serve temporarily on the *Kildonan Castle*. They arrived a week later, and conditions at Salonika were very different from those at Lemnos. The quality of food and living and working conditions were certainly better, although gastrointestinal ailments continued to be common, as were malaria and diphtheria.[131] According to historian Gerald Nicholson, 60 percent of the nurses serving at Salonika contracted malaria.[132] Seven of No. 4's nurses were invalided to England on the *Llandovery Castle* in September 1916. One of them, Lena Davis, recovered after being treated at the Moore Barracks Hospital and resumed nursing in No. 4, now in Basingstoke, but then contracted malaria again and died in February 1918.[133]

No. 4 nurses were also hospitalized in March 1917 suffering from "nervous debility," and between April and July "significant numbers" of them, including their matron, Annie Jane Hartley, were sent to a Red Cross convalescent home, and others were returned to England.[134] Hartley was briefly succeeded by Carolyn Viets, a Nova Scotian nurse who had served as matron of No. 2 CSH in France and received the Royal Red Cross 2nd Class in June 1916. She didn't last long, however, because she contracted diphtheria in November 1916 and was transferred to England in August 1917.

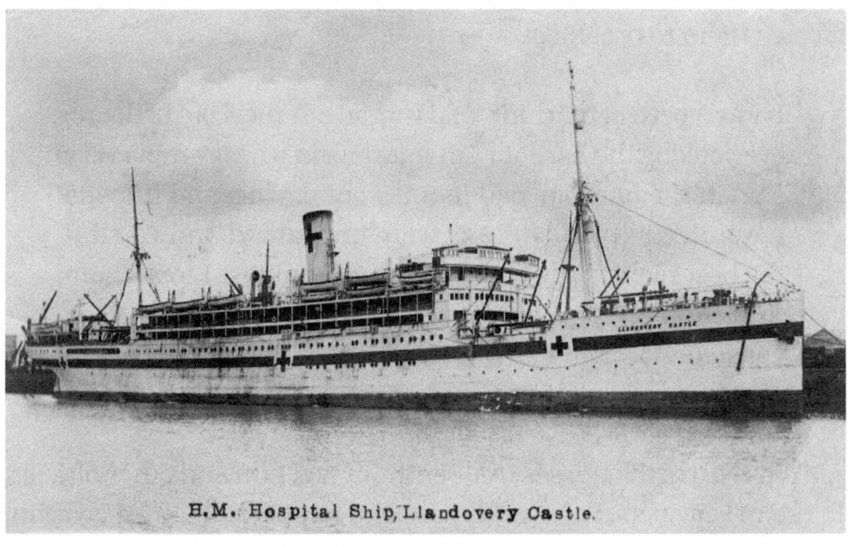

Hospital Ship HMHS *Llandovery Castle.* [NS ARCHIVES]

Mackenzie had nothing but praise for No. 4's nurses. In his opinion, "the person who does the most good in a Hospital like ours is the nursing Sister. The majority of the men do not need a great deal of attention from the physician or surgeon, except now and then, but all the time the Sister is looking after them and it makes so much difference to them.... We have an exceptionally good lot of nurses" and "they do an awful lot of good" despite the winter conditions which involved sleet and snow at times but also heavy rain that turned the camp into a "sea of mud."[135] He also noted that during an air raid the nurses were supposed to get into the "dugouts" but they "refused to leave the patients."[136]

Mackenzie's letters are particularly interesting because he relates how he and other officers mingled socially with the nurses when not on duty. On New Year's Eve, for example, when the nurses organized "an entertainment," they invited all medical staff to "go in masquerade" and the event was "very amusing" and "everybody was happy." He and other doctors soon got in the habit of taking nurses on hikes and picnics and playing bridge with them in their recreation tent. On one occasion he took "my six Sisters" to a restaurant and treated them to breakfast:

> It was a perfect morning, and we had our meal out of doors, overlooking the harbour. After last night's heavy rain every ship in the harbour had its sails out drying, and it made a wonderful picture. They were enchanted and voted it the best picnic they had had. After breakfast I took them to the top of the White Tower, a wonderful old Venetian construction, after which I took them to see the French pictures and then after some shopping we came home.[137]

In return, the nurses frequently invited him and other officers to their "very popular" weekly teas and suppers. On one occasion, "we had steak and fried potatoes and hot coffee—seven nurses and myself, then my plum pudding, for which one of the nurses had made some brandy sauce. I remained afterwards and helped them dry the dishes."[138] All in all, Mackenzie appears to have been popular with the nurses, and he clearly appreciated their work.

Little is known about No. 5 CGH, apparently because, according to Wagner, its records were "fragmentary."[139] Organized in Victoria, British Columbia, it was commanded by Dr. Edward Hart, a Nova

Scotian who was a general practitioner, city coroner, and was also active in the militia. In September 1915 he took the unit to England where it administered the Shorncliffe Military Hospital and therefore had no experience outside of England when it was sent to Salonika in December 1915.

Meanwhile, its seventy-one nurses remained in Cairo until February 1916.[140] Between March 1916 and July 1917, however, "significant numbers" of them were admitted to hospital or the British Red Cross Convalescent Home at Salonika, suffering from illness and "nervous debility."[141] Among them was Ethel Morrison, who was from Pictou but had moved with her parents to Victoria, British Columbia, in the late 1890s and was a graduate of the Vancouver General Hospital's School of Nursing. She had CAMC experience when she joined the CAMCNS in Victoria in September 1915, and after serving in No. 5 CGH at Salonika, she served in No. 1 CGH in France and England, was awarded the Royal Red Cross 2nd Class, and was twice mentioned in dispatches.

Meanwhile, No. 1 CSH had arrived at Salonika and appears to have struggled with the situation. Aside from the general conditions, many if not most of its nurses "vigorously disliked" their matron, Eleanor Charleson, who they not only described as a "self-absorbed incompetent" but also "expressed a deep distrust of her character, her motives," and her "pettiness and selfishness." They also thought she was unsociable and was hoping to get transferred back to England or France instead of helping her nurses to get transferred.[142] More disturbing was that at least three nurses—Laura Holland, Mildred Forbes and Helen Fowlds—thought she "was motivated more by concern for her personal reputation than altruist care of suffering patients."[143]

And yet, Charleson praised her nurses in October 1916 when they purchased rolled oats at exorbitant prices from local dealers so that their patients "may have porridge for breakfast" because "farinaceous food" was "important to their convalescence." She also praised the patients because, "like all the Tommies, they never complain, and thoroughly appreciate the Sisters, whose every effort is on their behalf." It also "speaks volumes for the efficiency of the unit" because most of patients arrived as "physical wrecks [and]... the death-rate was singularly low."[144]

Even so, No. 1's nurses thought Charleson was unagreeable. Her service record shows, however, that while serving in France, she had been mentioned in dispatches and was awarded the Royal Red Cross 2nd Class despite falling ill on several occasions. When she fell ill again in June 1917, she had to be invalided to England for a second time.

In October 1917 the three Canadian hospitals at Salonika were recalled to England. No. 1 CSH, redesignated No. 13 CGH, took over the Canadian military hospital at Hastings, No. 4 CGH took over the Canadian military hospital at Basingstoke, and No. 5 CGH took over the Canadian military hospital at Kirkdale. No. 3 CSH and No. 5 CSH, redesignated No. 7 CGH, had already been reposted to France in April 1916.

CHAPTER 3

The Home Front

Nova Scotia was the only province that was directly exposed to the war because it was the closest to Europe on the Atlantic Ocean. Its capital, Halifax, was the largest city in Eastern Canada and a major British and Canadian naval base and the headquarters of the Canadian army's Military District No. 6 (MD 6), from which most Canadian troops sailed to and from England during the war. Sydney, the second largest city in Nova Scotia and the centre of the province's coal and steel industry, was also important because its harbour also had a naval base that guarded the Gulf of St. Lawrence, and it was closer to England than Halifax.

By 1916, wounded men had begun arriving on hospital ships and fast liners like the *Olympic* at Halifax, because it was linked directly to central Canada by both sea and rail and also was well equipped with hospitals. The arrival of convalescent soldiers proved to be somewhat controversial, however, because the military authorities initially disembarked the seriously wounded ones onto small boats before docking at Pier 2, presumably to protect the general public from noticing the more disturbing cases. "Fortunately," as David Mossman has written, "a specific complaint registered by a local official, to the effect that even a sick cat shouldn't be treated like that, led to all future landings of wounded men being made after the ship docked."[145]

The result was that civic organizations began organizing garden parties, outings in automobiles and even harbour cruises. The YMCA and YWCA joined to form the Patriotic Service Battalion, whose mission was to provide "social entertainment for the soldier and sailor boys." Those who were bedridden were initially placed in the Cogswell Street Military Hospital (CMH), but when it was unable to accommodate the numbers, the overflow went to the naval hospital at the dockyard, the small army hospital at the Wellington Barracks on Gottingen Street, the Pier 2 Casualty Clearing Hospital, the CAMC Training Depot, and the former Admiralty House that had been converted into a hospital. By June 1918 there were four "battalions" in operation in the city. They even had a uniform: "the popular white middy...with the YWCA blue triangle on the sleeve."[146]

Halifax was not prepared, however, when it earned the unenviable distinction of being the only city in Canada to experience first-hand the dangers of modern warfare on the morning of December 6, 1917. At 9:05 am, when many people were already at work in the dockyards, factories and foundries, and others were on their way to work or school, two ships collided in the Narrows, the channel that linked the harbour with Bedford Basin. The *Imo*, a Norwegian tramp steamer under charter as a Belgian relief ship, was moving from the basin to the harbour en route to New York, while the *Mont Blanc*, a French-owned freighter, was moving from the harbour into the basin to join a convoy sailing to France.

The result was the greatest man-made explosion until atomic bombs were dropped on Japan in 1945, killing at least 1,946 men, women and children and injuring another 8,000, flattening the north end of the city and the adjacent Dartmouth area, leaving some 25,000 people homeless or without adequate shelter. Nurse Irene Thompson undoubtedly spoke for all overseas nurses when she wrote on the 8th that "all the people from there are crazy with anxiety."[147]

The CAMC supplied 56 doctors and 136 nurses from ships in the harbour.[148] Another 153 doctors and more than 450 nurses from across the province, nearby provinces and the northeastern US flooded into the city to help out as well.[149] Among the first of them were Dr. George DeWitt of Wolfville, his daughter, Nellie DeWitt, who was a nurse, and her brother, Major Avery DeWitt, who had served overseas with the CAMC but was now the medical officer at Camp Aldershot. They were accompanied by two nurses, Georgina Miner and Jessie Parker.[150]

Lieutenant Colonel Dr. Frederick McKelvey Bell, the assistant director of medical services for MD 6, who had served overseas with No. 2 CSH, the first Canadian hospital to go to France, and had two-years' first-hand experience with destruction, later told a newspaper reporter that he "had never seen anything on the battlefront equal to the scenes of destruction that he witnessed in Halifax today."[151]

As shocking as this was, more shocking was the fact that only five months earlier, on August 1, the *Letitia*, a hospital ship that sailed regularly between Liverpool, England, and Halifax, had run aground in thick fog on the rocky ledges at the entrance to the harbour. Local naval vessels responded quickly and succeeded in evacuating everyone on board—the 74 hospital staff, 546 patients, and crew—with the exception of one man, who drowned while attempting to swim ashore. There was, of course, an inquiry and the pilot was found guilty of a gross error of judgment and was demoted. No lessons were learned, however, which largely explains why the explosion took place and proved to be as disastrous as it was.

The army responded immediately despite the heavy damage at the Wellington Barracks and the armoury. Lieutenant Colonel W. E. Thompson, a fifty-two-year-old Halifax lawyer who had been active for years in the 63rd Regiment and was adjutant general of MD 6, called in all available troops from their various posts and sent them out into the streets to look for injured people, help them get to places where they could receive medical treatment, help recover bodies, and try to find people who might still be alive in the rubble of their homes. Among the first to be deployed were 150 American men from the Imperial Recruits Depot, who were on parade in the armoury at the time. They marched down to the waterfront and worked all day, even though some of them had actually been injured in the explosion. Other troops from the armoury and the huts on the Common were ordered out immediately, and by one o'clock every man who could be spared from the 63rd and 66th Regiments and from the artillery manning the forts had joined them, searching for and rescuing people from the ruins of buildings, extinguishing fires, clearing and patrolling the streets, and furnishing guards where necessary.

It was not just the soldiers who pitched in to help the stricken city. As it happened, virtually the whole Royal Canadian Navy fleet was in harbour at the time, including not only the Halifax-based vessels but also the Sydney Patrol, which had just moved to Halifax for the winter months. Remarkably, none of their ships were badly damaged except for the *Niobe*, the navy's first warship, which was anchored at the dockyard very close to where the collision took place. There were also three British and two American ships in port, and they were quickly joined by two American troop transports returning from Europe, which changed course for Halifax when they spotted the huge black cloud on the horizon. On arrival the *Tacoma* transferred its medical officers and staff to the *Old Colony*, while equipment was transferred from the *Morrill* to set up operating rooms and provided 250 men to help patrol the streets.

The situation was desperate. The Pier 2 Casualty Clearing Hospital and the Rockhead Military Hospital had both been destroyed, and the Cogswell Street Military Hospital had been badly damaged, while the naval hospital had been damaged but could carry on, although the staff and cadets of the naval school, which had shared the naval hospital building, had to be sent to the military college in Kingston, Ontario.[152] Alice Boutin, one of the two nurses at the naval hospital, was seriously wounded, but Frances Young transferred to the American ship *Old Colony*, which had been in drydock for repairs and was converted into a hospital ship capable of caring for 150 patients. Meanwhile, the CAMC Training Depot and the former Admiralty House were converted into small hospitals that were able to treat injured in the hours after the explosion.[153]

More importantly, the VGH, the Halifax Infirmary, the Salvation Army Maternity Hospital and Children's Home, the Nova Scotia Hospital at Woodside, and the Rockhead Infectious Diseases Hospital on Gottingen Street were swamped with casualties. Luckily, the new Camp Hill Hospital on Robie Street had just been completed, although it was not yet fully staffed or furnished. It was soon "jammed with badly hurt civilians, with patients lying on the beds, under the beds, even in the halls. The hard-driven doctors and nurses could only patch up those who were able to walk and send them home."[154]

Temporary treatment centres were also improvised at the armoury, the YMCA's gymnasium on Barrington Street, St. Mary's College,[155] the Pine Hill Presbyterian College, the Halifax Ladies College on Pleasant Street, the Oxford School on North Street, and the Waegwoltic Club. The private hospitals of Dr. Daniel Parker, Dr. Anthony Mader, and Dr. Clement Ligoure—the first Black physician to practise in Nova Scotia—were utilized as well. One unique convalescent hospital that had already been donated to the Military Hospitals Commission in 1916 was the mansion of William and Emily Clayton in Rockingham, a suburb of Halifax that had not been damaged by the explosion. Their large clothing factory was totally destroyed, however, because it was situated where Scotia Square is now.[156]

Many people fled to Armdale, and some kept going until they reached the woods beyond Dutch Village Road. A few hours later soldiers came and told them that they could return home, but that night there was a howling blizzard. Perhaps even worse, at least for Thomas Raddall, was that soldiers asked him to show them around the basement of Chebucto Road School, which he attended, only to discover that it was going to be used as the emergency morgue. When he got home and his mother asked what the soldiers had wanted him for, "I didn't care to say. I wanted to get those nightmare pictures out of my mind."[157]

Dartmouth tends to be ignored in accounts of the explosion, but it was devastated as well. It was a smaller community with a smaller population, but important industries such as the ropeworks on Wyse Road, Starr Manufacturing's rolling mill and Army & Navy Brewery building were destroyed. So too was the Mi'kmaw village at Turtle Grove which had been scheduled to move to Albro Lake in November. Historian Harry Chapman summed it up succinctly: "North Dartmouth was in shambles," and the downtown core was "awash in a sea of broken glass, rubble and debris."[158] Soldiers and voluntary firefighters were called out to help fight fires, to rescue people trapped in the rubble, and to urge everyone to vacate their homes at least temporarily.

Many people gathered in public spaces like Victoria Park, Notting Park, the Dartmouth Common and Silvers Hill, where they waited hopefully for their wounds to be treated or to be transported to hospital while the dead were loaded onto carts or trucks and taken to either of the town's two undertakers. Dr. Daniel Parker turned his home on Pleasant Street into a makeshift hospital, as did Henry Rosenburg on Crichton Avenue. Greenvale School became a medical aid station, and the Nova Scotia Hospital at Woodside, although damaged, was able to take in 150 patients. Remarkably, the ferries were still functional—there were no bridges yet—and worked all night, transporting victims to hospitals in Halifax and taking rescue workers, equipment and supplies to Dartmouth.[159]

Meanwhile, cities and towns in the Maritimes also sent doctors and nurses and offered temporary housing and food relief for the survivors. Sydney sent fourteen doctors and twenty-one nurses, while also welcoming patients in its military and civilian hospitals. Undertakers also came in from around the province and farther afield. Hundreds of people were sent by train to Windsor, Truro, Bridgewater and Wolfville as well, where improvised hospitals were established in churches, schools and other facilities. One unexpected casualty of the explosion was Dr. Nathan Shacknove of Whitney Pier in Sydney. He returned home after helping out in Halifax for several days and died by suicide, reportedly after having "brooded over the disaster for several days."[160]

Prime Minister Robert Borden, who was, of course, a Nova Scotian, was en route from Charlottetown to Pictou in the final days of the 1917 election campaign when he heard about the disaster and went directly to Halifax, arriving "in the midst of one of the most terrible blizzards I ever experienced."[161] He immediately authorized $500,000 for urgent aid and next day met with Abraham Ratshesky, a Boston businessman and state senator representing Governor Samuel McCall, who had already assured Halifax Mayor Peter Martin that Massachusetts was "ready to go the limit in rendering every assistance you may be in need of."[162] Martin did not receive the telegram because the lines were down, but McCall went ahead and formed the Halifax Relief Expedition, then proceeded to organize a special train—donated by the Boston and Maine Railroad—to take doctors, nurses and supplies to Halifax. A public meeting at Faneuil Hall in Boston launched a fundraising campaign that raised $100,000 on the first day.

Colonel Bell converted Bellevue House on Spring Garden Road, formerly the residence of the commandants of British Armed Forces that had later been occupied by military doctors, into an emergency hospital for the Massachusetts' medical team of 30 doctors and 50 nurses headed by Dr. William Edwards Ladd, a prominent Boston physician and surgeon. Massachusetts also sent 13 medical professionals from its state guard, and Harvard University sent what was described as a complete hospital unit. Maine sent 110 doctors, plus nurses and other volunteers, the Rhode Island Red Cross sent 50 doctors, 53 nurses, and a pharmacist, and the New York Red Cross sent several trains with engineers, doctors, nurses, tools, lumber, medical supplies and 1,000 portable houses. Other relief trains began arriving from Maine, Philadelphia and Washington as well. The Halifax Ladies College became a hospital for the Maine team, St. Mary's College for the American Red Cross, and the Halifax Infirmary and Bellevue House both made room for the Rhode Island unit.[163] Captain Eugene O'Donnell of the US Steamboat Inspection Service in Boston organized a ship that sent supplies, including 25,000 blankets, and the US Army sent relief supplies including food, as well.

The people of Nova Scotia, and particularly Halifax, were astonished and gratified but probably not surprised by this extraordinary generosity on the part of their southern neighbours because Massachusetts was home to thousands of Nova Scotians who had crossed the border over the years seeking better economic opportunities. Indeed, most Nova Scotians—including Prime Minister Borden—could trace their ancestry to New Englanders who had moved north either as Planters in the 1750s or Loyalists during the American

Revolution. More recently, women had trained in nursing schools in New England, and when the Spanish influenza epidemic swept North America in 1918, thirty-three Nova Scotian nurses helped out in Massachusetts and twelve of them died.[164]

It didn't take long for news of the disaster to reach the troops in Europe, some of whom—especially those in the 25th and 85th Battalions and the Royal Canadian Regiment—were from Halifax. We can only imagine the alarm caused by the news, which was limited by the fact that communications with Halifax were cut off for days. The army made every effort to obtain reliable information for families, and most men remained on duty. Inevitably, some learned that their families were safe while others had family and close relatives killed or badly injured. A few men were allowed to return home on compassionate leave, after which they were either discharged or reassigned as instructors at Camp Aldershot.

Massachusetts' generosity did not end in 1918. Upon their return home, many of the people involved in the relief effort formed the Halifax-Massachusetts Relief Associates, who raised $716,000 to improve the lives of survivors and general health conditions in the city. Nova Scotia also sent Boston a giant Christmas tree as a special offering of thanks in December 1918. The gesture was not immediately repeated, but it was revived in 1971 and continues to this day. How significant this annual gift is to the people of Boston is difficult to assess, but the process of selecting, cutting and shipping the tree to Boston continues to be very significant in Nova Scotia because it not only reminds people of the terrible disaster that took place in December 1917, but it also constitutes a unique bond of kinship between the two communities.

CHAPTER 4

Victory at Last

When Germany launched Operation Michael in March 1918, its last desperate offensive on the Western Front, hoping to end the war before the United States joined the Allies, its army broke through the allied lines and got close to Saint-Omer, the British army headquarters, which was shelled and attacked by air raids. No. 7 CSH and No. 9 CSH were evacuated to nearby Étaples, a major railway centre where several other military hospitals, including No. 1 CGH, were already situated. They arrived just in time for the infamous German air raid that took place on May 18–19, 1918. Matron-in-Chief Macdonald had assured McCarthy in October 1917 that "every Nurse in the Field is not only prepared but willing to make the great sacrifice and to share equal risks with the men in the trenches,"[165] and they were put to the test when thirty German aircraft attacked Étaples, perhaps intending to destroy the train station and railyards but also hitting the nearby hospitals.

No. 1 CGH's war diary provides a detailed account of the event, which began as enemy aircraft "came over the camp in large numbers" at 10:00 P.M., when the hospital was "wrapt in slumber." They began by dropping incendiary and high explosive bombs on the sleeping quarters of the personnel, turning them into "a conflagration and charnel house of dead and wounded men. Bombs were also dropped on the Officers' and Sisters' quarters," which were "completely wrecked.... While the work of receiving the wounded was going on, the enemy continued to drop bombs. Two of the hospital wards received direct hits and patients were killed and wounded." Nurses and officers who had escaped injury immediately attended to the needs of those who had been hit, and while the raid was in progress, the operating room staff were working on the cases injured.[166]

Of all the hospitals that were bombed in the raid, No. 1 CGH suffered the most casualties: sixty-six killed and seventy-three injured.[167] Among the dead were three nurses—Margaret Lowe, Katherine Macdonald and Gladys Wake—the first Canadian nurses to die in action in the war. Matron Edith Campbell specifically reported the "gallantry and devotion to duty" of Lottie Urquhart, a nurse from New Glasgow, Nova Scotia, who, when the bombs fell on her ward, "regardless of danger, attended to the wounded. Her courage and devotion were an inspiring example to all."[168] Because the hospital was now in no condition to receive patients, its personnel were temporarily transferred, and patients were moved to other hospitals in the

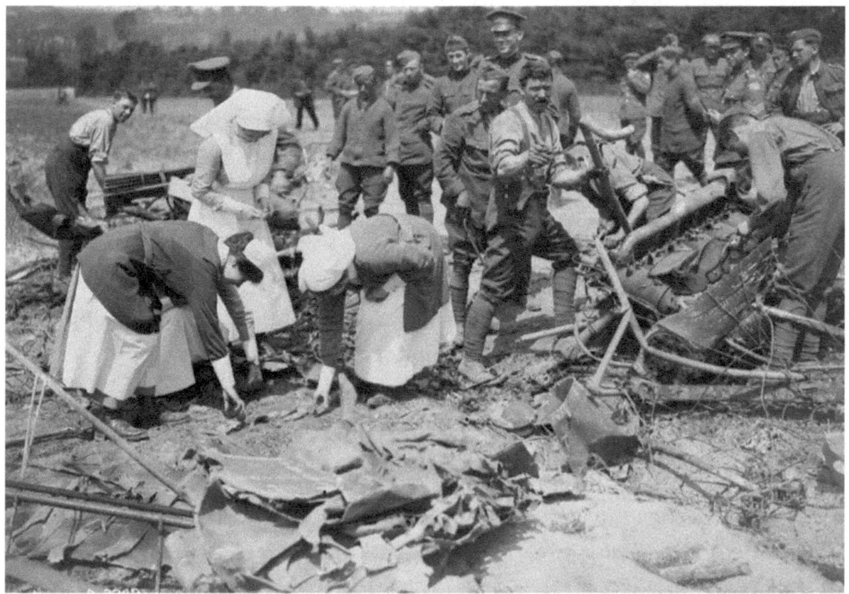

Canadian nurses viewing the remains of a German bomber that destroyed their hospital, June 1918. [CANADA, DEPT. OF NATIONAL DEFENCE/LIBRARY AND ARCHIVES CANADA]

area. In July it moved from Étaples to Trouville, where it remained until the end of the war.

No. 7 CSH experienced only "shrapnel...falling on the roof in showers," according to Nurse Irene Thompson,[169] but three men—Fred Laidlaw, an orderly from Wittenburg, Colchester County, and two patients—were killed, and Major Dr. E. V. Hogan, who had succeeded Dr. John Stewart in command, was wounded.[170] A few days later a second raid took place when, according to Thompson, "the Hun came over about 8:30 P.M. and stayed until about midnight" when "a very critical operation was taking place...Two doctors [were] operating while the bombs were dropping all around us" but only "one bomb dropped just outside our ward. The men in my ward [remained] very calm."[171] The only impact on the nurses was that those not on night duty had to "get away and sleep in the woods about three miles from [t]here."[172]

Meanwhile, No. 9 CSH had just moved to Étaples on May 9 and was not yet receiving patients when the attack took place. Even so, its war diary reported that German aircraft dropped seven bombs, three on the hospital and four among the tents of its personnel, killing Dr. William Fielding McIsaac of Antigonish and two orderlies, Horace MacMillan of Isaacs Harbour, Guysborough, and William Taylor of Toronto, Ontario, who had served in the composite battalion at Halifax. Twelve other personnel were wounded.[173]

More shocking, another air raid took place on the night of May 29–30 at Doullens, southwest of Étaples, where No. 3 CSH had been situated since November 1916. According to its war diary, "the night was clear and the moon was shining," and "red crosses on its buildings were "very visible" when a German aircraft began attacking the hospital just after midnight. It was "longer and in some ways more terrifying" than the raid on Étaples on the 31st because the planes flew low and fired their machine guns, "lasting two and a half hours, with flares, which had been dropped to light up the area and return anti-aircraft fire."[174] Three surgical teams were on duty that night, but two had completed their operations and had gone for their midnight meal. The third team was not so lucky. As it was finishing its operation, all—the patient, the doctors, nurses, orderlies and stretcher bearers—died. None of them were Nova Scotians although the surgeon, Dr. Ethelbert "Edward" Meek was born in Truro. His assistant, who is never mentioned in accounts of this event, was Dr. A. P. H. Sage, an American surgeon from Tennessee who had been attached to the RAMC and posted to No. 3. The three nurses were Dorothy Baldwin, Agnes MacPherson and Eden Pringle.[175]

Matron Edith Campbell of No. 1 CGH praised her nurses for their "splendid work" because this raid "was much harder to bear than the others, with much greater strain on both the nursing sisters and officers on duty."[176] When the Canadian government recommended that she and fifteen nurses be awarded the Military Cross for their courageous action under enemy fire, British authorities balked because the Canadian nurses were the only military nurses in the Commonwealth that had officer status, and they had to be content with the Military Medal.[177]

While Operation Michael gained the German forces more of France's territories, it failed to capture any strategic settlements. Subsequent German operations led to the Allies' counterattack that started the Hundred Days Offensive, which turned the tide of the war and cemented the Allies' victory.

It's worth noting too that five Nova Scotian doctors also died in service. Dr. Kenneth MacCuish of St. Peters, Richmond County, who had practised in Glace Bay and taught at St. Joseph's Hospital, served in No. 9 Field Ambulance and was killed at Passchendaele in October 1917. Dr. William Fielding McIsaac and Dr. Ethelbert Meek were killed in May 1918, and Dr. Thomas Howard MacDonald of Port Hawkesbury, who commanded the *Llandovery Castle* hospital ship, died when it was sunk in June 1918.

Dr. Walter MacLean, who was from Alberta but was a graduate of Dalhousie University's medical school, died when German aircraft bombed No. 1 CCCS at Zuydcoote in November 1918. Remarkably, Dr. MacLean practiced in Glace Bay with Dr. MacCuish and Dr. Donald MacLeod, who had joined No. 7 CSH in 1915 and also served in No. 1 CCCS. MacCuish's wife was a nurse who served overseas, and in

1921 MacLeod married Margaret Stewart, also a nurse who had served overseas.

At the same time the weary soldiers were anxious to get home, but organizing the shipping proved to be a problem in the spring of 1919. Frustration and anger were prevalent because of poor management and influenza at Kinmel Park, a demobilization camp in Wales occupied by some 15,000 men served by No. 9 CGH and sixteen Nova Scotian nurses. Seventy-eight men and one nurse died from influenza. Rebecca MacIntosh, who was from Pleasant Bay, Cape Breton, rests in St. Margaret's churchyard in the nearby village of Bodelwyddan.

As the Allied forces pushed eastward, nurses found themselves having to encounter not only prisoners of war but also large numbers of civilians, many of whom were casualties or suffering from starvation. According to Hallett, "some British and Canadian surgical teams had been loaned to French military hospitals that had, traditionally, always been more ready to treat civilians," and one surgical team from No. 4 CCCS "worked at an operating theatre in Arras, caring for large numbers of wounded and gassed civilians. It was found that many elderly patients had been lying in cellars, sheltering from the fighting for several weeks, and were suffering from severe pressure sores."[178]

Over the years different figures have been given for how many nurses died in the war. Part of the problem is that, with respect to soldiers, some only count those who died during the war while others include those who died not long after as a result of injuries received during the war. The government's cut-off date for determining Canada's war dead was August 31, 1921, but Canada's *Book of Remembrance* includes those who died up to April 30, 1922.[179] That is the date used in this study. Andrew Macphail claimed in 1925 that thirty-nine Canadian nurses had died in the war[180] but when the memorial panel honouring Canada's military nurses was mounted in the Centre Block of the parliament building in 1926, the names of eight nurses who died while serving in the QAIMNS and six others who died while serving in the United States Army Nurse

Corps were added, raising the total to fifty-three, twelve of whom were Nova Scotians.[181]

The accepted figure today, presumably based on Dianne Dodd's research, is sixty-one, but she includes two women, Beatrice Bartlett and Dorothy Pearson Twist, who died in England in the influenza epidemic and are included on the Canadian Virtual War Memorial but were VADs, not trained nurses.[182] Meanwhile, Neil MacLean, a Nova Scotian nurse, is not listed on the nurses' memorial panel in the parliament building or included in Dodd's list even though he was killed in action, presumably because he and other male nurses were only allowed to serve as stretcher bearers and orderlies.

Macphail reminds us that "every one" of the 761,635 wounded or ill Canadians, thousands of Allied soldiers and untold numbers of prisoners of war and civilians "passed through the hands of a CAMC nursing sister," and historian Desmond Morton points out that "93 per cent of those who reached treatment survived their wounds."[183] These figures explain why Canadian nurses received 438 honours: 64 first class Royal Red Crosses and 253 second class Royal Red Crosses, 109 mentions in dispatches, 9 Military Medals, 2 OBEs and 1 Royal Victorian Order medal.[184]

And yet, when a memorial in the parliament buildings to honour the nurses who served in the war was proposed, the government resisted the idea, perhaps not unreasonably because a previous government had already included an impressive memorial to those who had died while serving in the war in the new Peace Tower built after the 1916 fire in the parliament building. Prime Minister W. L. Mackenzie King finally relented in 1925 but insisted, perhaps with an eye on Quebec, that it honour the history of Canadian nurses generally. That is why the text on the memorial includes the somewhat irrelevant statement that it perpetuates "a noble tradition in the relations of the Old World and the New" and exemplifies "an heroic service embracing three centuries of Canadian history."

The government also required that the nurses, through their associations, cover the $32,000 cost of the memorial. They did so but made clear in the text that it had been "erected by the nurses

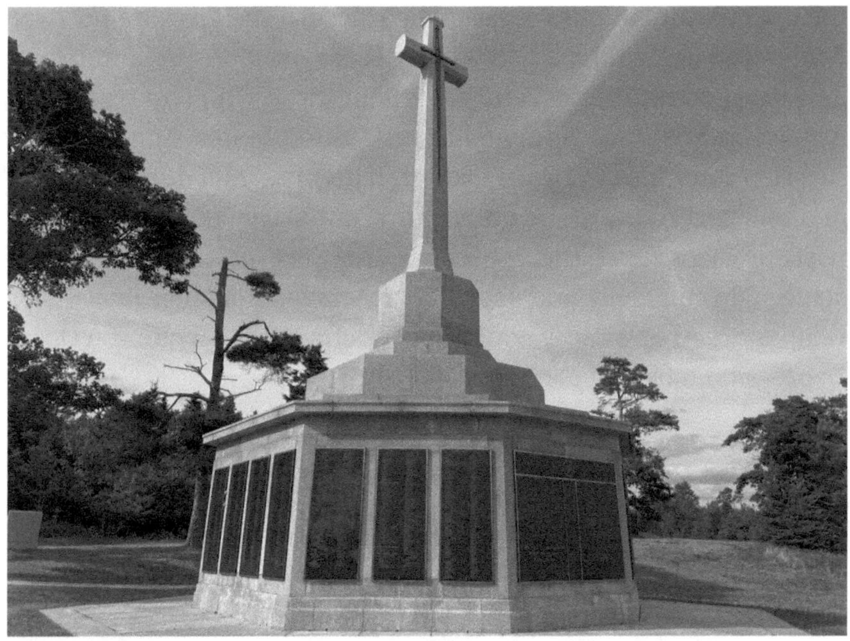

The Halifax Memorial in Point Pleasant Park in Halifax, built by the Commonwealth War Graves Commission. It commemorates Canadian and Newfoundland sailors, soldiers, and nurses who lost their lives in the First and Second World Wars. [CONTRIBUTED]

of Canada in remembrance of their sisters who gave their lives in the Great War, 1914–1918."[185] By comparison, York Minster in Yorkshire unveiled the names of all the nurses from throughout the Commonwealth who had died in the war on its famed Five Sisters stained windows.[186]

As much as veterans, including nurses, were generally honoured in the postwar years, many of them struggled to adjust in the transition from wartime to life in the new world. Many returned to their pre-war jobs if they were available, while others found it difficult to find employment. Men often found it more difficult to return to their old jobs, if they still existed, especially if they had been replaced by women who were paid lower wages. Some nurses returned to nursing in their home communities and families, of course, while others transferred into military convalescent hospitals. Others still took the opportunity to pursue related careers in the growing postwar field of public health, which offered them positions in both urban and rural communities, and several of those who had trained in American hospitals returned to the United States. Many nurses married veterans or physicians whom they had met during the war or afterward. At the same time, many unmarried nurses found the postwar years very difficult because they were, of course, older and struggled financially and socially, especially after their parents or relatives died or simply could not be supportive, when the Great Depression took place in 1930.[187]

Database

1. Allan, Ann Doctor (1882–1962). Born in Perth, Scotland, d/o James and Jessie (Calder) Allan, she emigrated to Nova Scotia in 1908 and was nursing in a hospital in Regina when she returned to Halifax and worked in the CMH. She joined the CAMCNS in Halifax in September 1914, naming Mrs. D. Campbell, 64 Almon Street, Halifax, as next of kin (NOK). She was posted to No. 2 CGH at Valcartier and went overseas with the first contingent on the *Franconia*. She also served in No. 1 CCCS, No. 1 CGH and No. 16 CGH, was mentioned in dispatches in June 1916, and was awarded the Royal Red Cross 2nd Class in January 1917. She was struck off service (SOS) in August 1919 and nursed at the Sydney City Hospital in 1925 and later in the Kentville sanatorium until retiring in Windsor, Hants County, in 1945.
2. Allen, Adruenna. *See* Tupper, Adruenna.
3. Anderson, Edith Crockett (1880–1953). Born in Rivière-du-Loup, Quebec, d/o Thomas and Elizabeth (Seaton) Crockett and wife of Dr. Charles Willoughby Anderson, a physician who was born in Halifax but taught medicine at McGill University. When he joined No. 1 CGH in October 1916 with the rank of captain, Edith, who was nursing in Halifax and had CAMC experience, accompanied him and joined the CAMCNS in London. He served in hospitals in England, and she served in No. 3 CGH and No. 15 CGH. When he resigned his commission in October 1917, possibly for health reasons, she resigned as well, and they returned home. Shortly afterward, they moved to Los Angeles.
4. Anderson, Minerva Blanche (1889–1981). Born in Big Baddeck, Victoria County, d/o Alexander and Susan (Archibald) Anderson, she was a graduate of the RVH School of Nursing and nursed there and had CAMC experience when she joined the CAMCNS in April 1917. She served with No. 4 CGH at Basingstoke, No. 10 CGH at Brighton and No. 3 CGH at Boulogne. She returned to Canada in March 1919 and was director of nurses at the

Sydney City Hospital for many years. Her three brothers, Percival, James, and Daniel Anderson, served overseas in the 85th Battalion. Percival and James were officers, and both received the Military Cross, but Percival was killed at Passchendaele.

5. Anderson, Robita (1894–1980). Born in Dominion, Cape Breton, d/o Robert and Maria (MacRury) Anderson, Halifax, she was nursing in Halifax and had two months' CAMC experience when she joined the CAMCNS in July 1918, claiming to have been born in 1896. She served in Halifax with the MD 6 Training Depot and CMH, where she met Dr. Clarence Thorne, a graduate of the VGH medical school and a graduate physician-scientist (MDCM) of McGill University who had been conscripted in June 1918 and served in CHH. Following their marriage in April 1919, she was SOS in June 1919. They subsequently moved to Saskatoon.

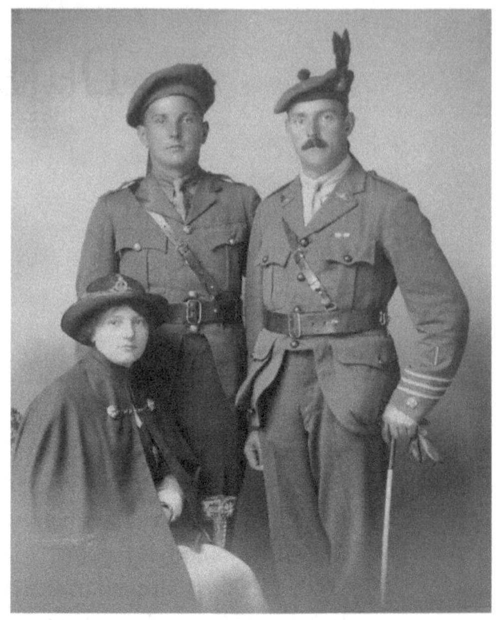

Minerva Blanche Anderson with her brothers, James Archibald (Archie) on the left and Percival on the right. Minerva is dressed in the uniform of a nursing sister in the Canadian Army Medical Corps. Her brothers were both officers in the 85th Battalion (Nova Scotia Highlanders). [ROBERT MACLELLAN COLLECTION, CAPE BRETON MILITARY HISTORY COLLECTIONS]

6. Andrews, Edyth Elizabeth (1887–1965). Born in Halifax, Halifax County, d/o George and Mary Flawn, Halifax, and wife (1901) of Charles Avener Andrews, Mahone Bay, a blacksmith, then a hotel keeper. Charles had enlisted in the 40th Battalion in 1915, was transferred into the 236th Battalion but was found to be physically unfit and discharged in May 1917. She had eight months' CAMC experience and joined the CAMCNS in July 1918. She reverted to the CAMC and served with the MD 6 Training Depot and CHH until being SOS in February 1919. They and their two children then moved to Liverpool, Queens County, where she nursed until 1947.

7. Archard, Sarah Ann "Sadie" (1883–1964). Born in Halifax, Halifax County, d/o Alfred and Margaret (Campbell) Archard, Halifax. Her father was a British soldier stationed at the Halifax garrison until becoming a dental

technician in 1910, and her mother was from Hunters Mountain, Cape Breton. Sarah was a 1914 graduate of the VGH School of Nursing and was night supervisor of nurses at the VGH until joining the CAMCNS in October 1915. She served in No. 7 CSH and briefly in the CEF Forestry Corps at Menton, France. She was awarded the Royal Red Cross 2nd Class in 1919, the Queen of Belgium Medal, and was mentioned in dispatches. After being SOS in April 1919, she went to New York and wrote examinations that qualified her as a registered nurse, a designation not yet available in Canada. She was appointed superintendent of nurses at CHH, then superintendent of the VGH Nurses private pavilion, built in 1922 to house the Departments of Neurosurgery and Psychiatry. An active member of the Canadian National Association of Trained Nurses, she was awarded the King George V Silver Jubilee Medal in 1935 and contributed to the passage of the act that incorporated the Graduate Nurses' Association of Nova Scotia. Following her death in 1964, the Sarah Archard Memorial Fund was established to assist VGH graduates in financial need, and in 2009 she was posthumously awarded the College of Registered Nurses of Nova Scotia Centennial Award of Distinction. Her brother, Edwin Archard, was conscripted in May 1918 and posted to the MD 6 Depot Battalion but immediately deserted and was SOS in March 1919.

8. Archibald, Cora Peters (1881–1956). Born in Truro, Colchester County, d/o Peter, an architect, and Elizabeth "Libby" (Dunlop) Archibald, she may have been related to Dr. Edward Archibald, a Montreal physician, s/o John Sprott Archibald, born in Musquodoboit, Nova Scotia, who had moved to Montreal in the 1860s and became a prominent lawyer and judge. Dr. Archibald joined the CAMC in October 1914 and served briefly in No. 3 CGH. Cora attended the Acadia University Seminary (collegiate course) and was a 1909 graduate of the RVH School of Nursing in Montreal. She was nursing at the Quebec Military Hospital when she joined the CAMCNS in May 1915. She served initially with No. 2 British Stationary Hospital but then transferred to No. 3 CGH. She also served with the RAMC No. 11 Stationary Hospital, the Canadian Forestry Corps Hospital at Lajoux and No. 16 CGH, until being SOS in May 1919. She subsequently nursed in Montreal but retired to Truro. Three brothers also served in the war: Captain Maxwell Stanfield Eaton Archibald served in the RAF and died of wounds in May 1918, Thomas Robert Archibald served overseas in the Canadian Forestry Corps in 1917–18, and Walter Gordon Archibald served overseas with the 36th Battery, Canadian Field Artillery from 1916 to 1919.

9. Bain, Margaret Winifred (1891–1970). Born in Saint-Raymond, Quebec, d/o James and Louise (Ross) Bain, Bridgewater, Lunenburg County. Her

father was born in Halifax but had moved to Quebec as a railway executive until transferring to Bridgewater, Lunenburg County, where he was superintendent of the Halifax and Southwestern Railway. Margaret attended the Acadia University Seminary (collegiate course) and had eight months' CAMC experience in Halifax and Sydney when she joined the CAMCNS in June 1918. She served in No. 11 CGH at Shorncliffe and No. 15 CGH, formerly the DCRC, a facility lent by Waldorf Astor, the American millionaire, on his estate, Cliveden, at Taplow, where the first hospital wards were in a closed tennis court. She contracted influenza in October 1918 and was SOS in February 1919. She married Cyril Gorham, a prominent businessman, and they lived in Halifax. After his death in 1962, she moved to Toronto to live with a sister. Her brother, Charles Bain, was a medical student at the VGH when he was conscripted in June 1918. He served at Camp Aldershot and was SOS in November 1918.

10. Barnaby, Agnes Gertrude (1885–1948). Born in Louisbourg, Cape Breton, d/o Dr. Clarence and Margaret (Hanley) (deceased)[188] Barnaby, Halifax, she was a 1912 graduate of the VGH School of Nursing, was night supervisor at the VGH and had a year's CAMC experience when she shaved four years off her date of birth and joined the CAMCNS in July 1918. She served at the MD 6 Training Depot and the CMH until falling ill and was SOS in March 1919. She continued nursing in Halifax until retiring in 1934.

11. Barnes, Ellen Caroline (1888–1982). Born in Sleaford, Lincolnshire, England, d/o Rev. Charles and Ellen (Mellor) Barnes, she was a nurse living with her parents in Dartmouth when she joined the CAMCNS in May 1917. She served briefly at No. 15 CGH (DCRC) Hospital, then fell ill and returned to Halifax in February 1918 for treatment at CHH. In April 1918 she married Charles Burdick, an American sailor from Michigan. They subsequently moved to New York and later to Snohomish, Washington.

12. Bauld, Muriel Hazel (1886–1987).[189] Born in Halifax, Halifax County, d/o William and Elizabeth "Bessie" (Bauld) Bauld, she joined the CAMCNS in July 1915, but her service file contains no information other than noting that she resigned in May 1917, presumably because she was about to marry William Coates Borrett (1894–1983), a son of Major W. J. Borrett, a British officer serving with the Royal Garrison Artillery in Halifax. He joined the regiment with the rank of captain and served in England from September to November 1918. After the war he managed CHNS, Nova Scotia's first radio station, and for several years broadcast a series called *Tales Told Under the Old Town Clock* that featured stories about Nova Scotian history. They were published by Ryerson Press, titled as *Tales Told Under the Old Town Clock* in 1942 and as *More Tales Told Under the Old Town Clock* in

1943. After his retirement from broadcasting, he commanded the Nova Scotia Division of the Canadian Corps of Commissionaires and oversaw the restoration of Citadel Hill, serving as honorary superintendent of the national historic site.

13. Bayer, Gladys Fuller (1889–1970). Born in Meaghers Grant, Halifax County, d/o James and Mary Ellen (Fuller) Bayer (deceased), she was nursing there and had CAMC experience when she joined the CAMCNS in Halifax in May 1917. She served in No. 8 CSH, No. 13 CGH and No. 16 CGH and was SOS in September 1919. In 1919 she married Thomas Henry McKillip, a Toronto physician who had joined the CAMC at Valcartier in September 1914, received the Distinguished Service Order (DSO) in June 1915 and rose to the rank of lieutenant colonel in London, Ontario. They lived in Toronto until moving to Nakina, Algoma County, Ontario, from 1931 to 1948, then moved to Vancouver.

14. Beairsto, Mary Keir (1883–1969). Born in Yarmouth, Yarmouth County, d/o Rev. John Keir (deceased) and Jane (Barnes) Beairsto. The family moved to Glassville, New Brunswick, but when her father died in 1912, Mary moved with her mother and siblings to Amherst, Cumberland County. It's not known where Mary trained, but it may have been in Halifax. She nursed in the Rockhead Military Hospital from 1916 until July 1918, when she joined the CAMCNS and served in the MD 6 Training Depot, the PEI Military Convalescent Hospital, and CHH and subsidiary facilities in Halifax. In July 1919 she contracted tuberculosis and was treated at the Nova Scotia Sanatorium until 1921. She then lived with her mother and four siblings on a farm in St. Mary's, New Brunswick, describing herself in the 1921 census as a "cook nurse." In 1931 she and her mother were living there alone. They are buried with her father in the Fredericton Rural Cemetery.

15. Benjamin, Vera Louise (1886–1974). Born in Bridgewater, Lunenburg County, d/o Daniel and Adelia (Manning) Benjamin (later Keefler), she was a graduate of the Massachusetts General Hospital School of Nursing and served in RAMC No. 22 General Hospital at Étaples in France with the Harvard Surgical Unit, which was staffed by American personnel from Harvard University.[190] In September 1916 she transferred into the CAMCNS, reducing her age by three years, and served with the DCRC, No. 7 CGH, the Granville Canadian Special (Convalescent) Hospital at Buxton, and No. 9 CGH when it was stationed at the Canadian Demobilization Camp at Kinmel Park in Wales from December 1918 to June 1919. In 1920 she married William Feindel, a merchant from Middleton who had settled in Bridgewater, and after his death in 1926, returned to nursing at CHH until retiring to Bridgewater, living with her sister, Lena (Benjamin) Davison, and died there.

16. Benvie, Ada (1883–1971). Born in Centre Musquodoboit, Halifax County, d/o James and Annie (Grant) Benvie, she was a 1909 graduate of the VGH School of Nursing and was nursing in Montreal and had CAMC experience when she joined the CAMCNS in Montreal in June 1915 and served in No. 2 CGH at Le Tréport and No. 2 CCCS until falling ill and being treated in London in December 1917. She then served with Granville Canadian Special Hospital at Buxton from June 1915 to May 1919, when she was SOS and returned to Halifax and served at CHH and the CMH until February 1920. She trained to be a public health nurse at the University of British Columbia, graduating in 1922 and lived in Duncan, Victoria, and Vancouver. Her brother, Augustus French Benvie, enlisted in the 17th Battalion in September 1914 but served in the Princess Patricia's Canadian Light Infantry and was killed in June 1916.
17. Bissett, Barbara Beatrice (1894–1989). Born in Cardigan, PEI, d/o Henry (deceased) and Emma (Norton) Bissett, who had moved to Windsor, Hants County. She was a 1917 graduate of the Newport Hospital School of Nursing in Rhode Island. She was living in Halifax and had six weeks' CAMC experience when she joined the CAMCNS in August 1918. She served in CHH and as principal matron for the MD 6 Training Depot until being SOS in August 1919. In 1921 she was supervisor of nurses at the Wellesley Hospital, Toronto, but was nursing in Windsor, Hants County, when she married Gerald Percy Strong in 1923 and was still there in 1929. Her brother, William Bissett, served with the 1st Royal Canadian Garrison Artillery in Halifax but died in Windsor, Hants County, in 1916.
18. Black, Amy Isobel (1882–1971). Born in Amherst, Cumberland County, d/o Joshua Hiram and Mary Elizabeth (Smith) Black (deceased), she had CAMC experience and was nursing in Nanaimo, BC, when she travelled to London, England, in September 1915 and joined the CAMCNS, naming her brother, Percy Black, as NOK. She served in No. 5 CGH, No. 2 CGH, the DCRC, No. 1 CGH, No. 9 CGH and No. 13 CGH before returning to Halifax where she nursed in CHH and the CMH. She was SOS in 1920 and returned to Amherst and in 1921, was living with her brother, Norman Black. She was not nursing, although her death certificate states that she nursed until 1931. Her father had represented Cumberland County in the House of Assembly from 1874 to 1878 and was a member of the Legislative Council from 1879 to 1897. Her brother served as the MLA for Cumberland from 1925 to 1940 and was Minister of Highways, then served in the House of Commons from 1945 to 1953.
19. Blair, Frances Maitland. *See* Frew, Frances Maitland.

20. Blood, Alice Margaret (1894–1999). Born in Bourne, Lincolnshire, England, d/o Arthur and Margaret (Holdich) Blood, she studied nursing at St. Bartholomew's Hospital in London and joined the QAIMNS and served in No. 16 CGH at Orpington, England, where she met Dr. Hugh MacKinnon, a physician from East Side Lake Ainslie, Inverness County, who had joined No. 5 CSH in July 1915 as a captain and later major. They moved to Canada in July 1919 and married in Quebec in September 1920, then lived in Inverness, Berwick, and finally Halifax, where he died in 1974. She may have been the last surviving nurse from the First World War when she died in the Camp Hill Veterans' Wing of the Queen Elizabeth II Health Sciences Centre in 1999 at the age of 105. The gates to the CHH memorial garden are dedicated to her memory.

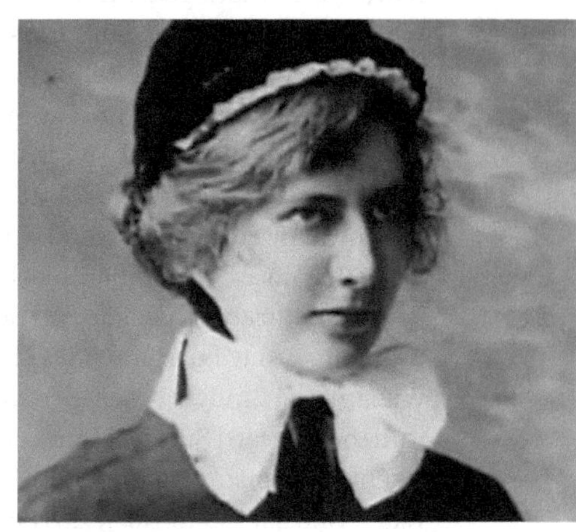

Alice Margaret Blood. [FINDAGRAVE.COM]

21. Boland, Florence Elizabeth (1889–1947). Born in Londonderry, Colchester County, d/o Daniel and Jane (Bell) Boland, Dartmouth, Halifax County, she had thirty months' CAMC experience when she joined the CAMCNS in January 1916. She served in the Rockhead Military Hospital, Pier 2 Casualty Clearing Hospital, and at the MD 6 Training Depot until May 1919, when she was SOS as physically unfit. In June 1919 she married Herbert Waugh, who had served as a lieutenant in the 6th Battalion, Canadian Garrison Regiment in Halifax. They later moved to Bridgeport, Connecticut.

22. Boutin, (Marie) Alice (1895–1983). Born in West Arichat, Richmond County, d/o François and Emelie Jane (LeBlanc) Boutin, she was one of the three medical staff serving at the Royal Canadian Naval Hospital on Gottingen Street when the Halifax Explosion took place on December 6, 1917. According to the Halifax *Morning Chronicle*, despite "a fractured rib and a dislocated shoulder," she and staff surgeon Joseph Rousseau "cared for the injured naval cadets and local civilians brought to the hospital until late in the evening...before she was relieved of her duty."[191] In fact, both of the hospital's nurses were on duty, but Frances Rand Young was only moderately injured, so she served on the US naval ship *Old Colony* and later published an account of her experiences. (*See* #309). Alice subsequently moved to Grimsby, Ontario, where she died.

23. Bowes, Christine "Christy" Ann (1880–1954). Born in Antigonish, Antigonish County, d/o Duncan and Margaret (McDonald) Chisholm and wife of David Bowes, who managed a hotel in Golden, BC, she was the housekeeper. When her husband died in 1915, she trained as a nurse and served in the Fairmont Military Hospital until joining the CAMCNS in February 1919. She served in the Shaughnessy Military Hospital until being SOS in April 1919 as "medically unfit." Her brother, Hugh Gillis Chisholm, a physician in Calgary, also joined the CAMC, serving in various hospitals including the Royal Air Force in England with the rank of captain, then major, until being diagnosed with tuberculosis and was SOS in May 1919.
24. Brennan, Elizabeth Cecilia. *See* Doyle, Elizabeth Cecilia.
25. Brennan, Emily Lorraine (1882–1955). Born in Pictou, Pictou County, d/o William and Emily (Fraser) Brennan, she had eleven months' experience with the Harvard Surgical Unit at RAMC No. 22 General Hospital at Étaples when she transferred into the CAMCNS in 1916, reducing her age by four years. She served in No. 5 CGH at Salonika until contracting dysentery, malaria, and tonsilitis and was invalided to England. She returned home in December 1917 for treatment at CHH and was SOS in August 1918. She married Edward Griffin, an insurance agent, in 1919, and they lived in Halifax, and she did not continue nursing.
26. Brenton, Grace Thurza (1889–1967). Born in Middle Stewiacke, Colchester County, d/o Robinson (deceased) and Margaret (Winton) Brenton, she went to England on her own and nursed at the DCRC in Taplow until transferring into the CAMCNS in September 1915, claiming to have CAMC experience and naming her brother, Walter Brenton, as NOK. She served in No. 5 CGH at Salonika from December 1915 to December 1916 when she fell ill. She returned to England, then home in January 1917, but then went back to England and served fourteen months at the DCRC, the Moore Barracks Hospital at Shorncliffe, later designated No. 11 CGH, and No. 15 CGH. She resigned in June 1918 to marry Major (Reginald) Frank Gambrill (1890–1975), a New Zealand army officer who served in the Wellington Regiment at Gallipoli and on the Western Front. They subsequently lived in Gisborne, New Zealand, where he was a lawyer and was active in the military, commanding the Hauraki Regiment from 1924 to 1926 and serving as Dominion vice-president of the Returned and Services Association.
27. Brock, Louise (1881–1930). Born in Burnt Islands, Newfoundland, d/o Philip and Ellen (Troke) Brock (both deceased). The family had moved to North Sydney, Cape Breton, in 1892, then to Saskatoon, Saskatchewan. Louise returned to Nova Scotia in 1910 and had a month's experience with the CMH in Halifax when she went to London and joined the CAMCNS in

February 1915, claiming to have been born in 1883. She served in No. 2 CSH at Boulogne, the Dardanelles and Salonika, and was mentioned in dispatches in October 1916 and was awarded the Royal Red Cross 2nd Class in June 1917. She served briefly as matron of No. 4 CGH at Westenhanger in September–October 1917 but resigned her commission and returned home in December 1917 to marry Sylvester Archibald, also a Nova Scotian. They lived in Saskatoon, and her letters and photos are housed in the University of Saskatchewan's archives.

28. Brown, Jessie Whidden. *See* Jaggard, Jessie Brown.

29. Burton, Mary Elizabeth (1878–1934). Born in Pictou, Pictou County, d/o William and Elizabeth (Webber) Burton, Halifax, she was an 1898 graduate of the VGH School of Nursing. She was nursing in Halifax and had two years' CAMC experience when she joined the CAMCNS in August 1918, naming her brother, William Henry Burton, Boston, as NOK. She served in the MD 6 Training Depot and CMH until being SOS in February 1919. In 1920 she married Harry Aarestrup, whose first wife, Mary's sister, Charlotte Burton, was killed with their eight-year-old son in the Halifax Explosion.

30. Calder, Janet "Jennie" Squair[192] (1883–1978). Born in Springville, Pictou County, d/o Frank and Christy (MacLean) Calder, she was a 1909 graduate of the VGH School of Nursing and briefly served as supervisor of nurses at a hospital in Chicago but was nursing at the Hamilton Hospital in North Sydney when she shaved three years off her date of birth and joined the CAMCNS in December 1915. She served in No. 7 CSH, RAMC No. 2 Stationary Hospital (Abbeville), the Kitchener Military Hospital (redesignated No. 10 CGH in September 1917) and the Canadian Officers' Hospital (London, Ontario), and was awarded the Royal Red Cross 2nd Class, the Queen of Belgium Medal, and was mentioned in dispatches. After being SOS in August 1919, she served as supervisor of nurses at the Sydney City Hospital and was later superintendent of nurses in a hospital in Alma, Michigan. She married John K. Campbell, a retired local businessman in Springville, and retired there.

31. Cameron, Anna May (1884–1962). Born in Big Island, Pictou County, d/o John (deceased) and Clotilda (Robertson) Cameron, she was a 1916 graduate of the VGH School of Nursing, had six weeks' experience with the King's College Cadet Corps in Windsor, Hants County, and shaved two years from her date of birth when she joined the CAMCNS in January 1917. She served overseas in No. 9 CSH, No. 12 CGH, No. 7 CGH, and the CAMC Casualty Company at Shorncliffe. In August 1918 she was transferred to Halifax and served in the CMH until requiring surgery for tonsilitis at CHH and was SOS in November 1918. A month later she married Charles Burpee

McMann, who was manager of the Pictou County Dairy in Stellarton. She did not continue nursing.

32. Cameron, Elizabeth Vena (1870–1961). Born in Lochaber, Antigonish County, d/o John Daniel and Margaret (Murray) Cameron. The family moved to Vancouver in 1901 after her father's death in 1893. She appears to have studied nursing in Montreal and reduced her age by at least seven years when she joined the CAMCNS there in June 1915. She served in No. 3 CSH, No. 5 CGH and No. 3 CCCS and was awarded the Royal Red Cross 2nd Class. She then served in the CAMC Casualty Company at Shorncliffe and the Canadian Red Cross Officers Hospital in London. After her mother died in 1918, she was SOS in July 1919 and returned to Vancouver.
33. Cameron, Josephine "Josie" Christine (1886–1971). Born in Bridgeville, Pictou County, d/o John (deceased) and Annabelle (McHardy) Cameron, she was a 1911 graduate of the VGH School of Nursing and was serving in the Dominion Iron and Steel Company Hospital in Sydney when she joined the CAMCNS in October 1915. She served in No. 7 CSH and No. 16 CGH until contracting influenza in 1918 and returned to Halifax in January 1919. She then served in CHH and was promoted to assistant matron until retiring in Bridgeville.
34. Cameron, Mary Lillian (1894–1956). Born in Canso, Guysborough County, d/o Frederick and Laura (Condon) Cameron, she was a 1917 graduate of a school of nursing in Montreal. She had experience with the 8th Field Ambulance there and served for nine months in a Montreal military hospital until joining the CAMCNS in May 1917. She went overseas in March 1918, serving in No. 4 CGH and briefly with No. 15 CGH and received the British War Medal. She returned to Canada in July 1919 and subsequently nursed in New York and Montreal as a public health nurse. In 1927 she married Colin Chisholm of Port Hood, a veteran who had served overseas in No. 7 Siege Battery, CFA, and the Royal Flying Corps. After the war he studied engineering at Queen's University and worked in Kirkland Lake, Ontario; Stirling, Cape Breton, and Beardmore, Ontario, until retiring in Montreal.
35. Campbell, Annie Mae (1891–?). Born in Springhill, Cumberland County, d/o Duncan and Hannah (McLennan) Campbell, she was living in Halifax and had eighteen months' CAMC experience when she joined the CAMCNS in April 1918. She served in No. 4 CGH in England and Salonika and No. 12 CGH at Bramshott Camp, returning home in July 1919. In 1921 she was nursing at the Highland View Hospital in Amherst, Cumberland County.
36. Campbell, Donalda Jean (1890–1980). Born in Big Island, Pictou County, d/o John (deceased) and Clotilda (Robertson) Cameron and wife of Lawrence Blair Campbell, she was a 1912 graduate of the VGH School of Nursing and

had CAMC militia experience when she joined the CAMCNS in Montreal in August 1916. She served in the DCRC, No. 9 CSH and No. 12 CGH until resigning and returning to Canada in December 1917. Lawrence Blair Campbell was a student with militia experience, living in Halifax when they married in March 1915 just before he enlisted in the CEF in April 1915. He served initially as a sergeant with the Canadian Cycle Corps and No. 3 Canadian Field Ambulance until returning home in April 1919. He became a clergyman, and they lived in Amherst and Stewiacke but later moved to Vernon, British Columbia.

37. Campbell, Jean Marion (1881–1960). Born in Glenelg, Guysborough County, d/o Samuel and Margaret (Archibald) Campbell, she was living in Halifax and had two years, eight months' CAMC militia experience when she joined the CAMCNS in July 1918. She served at the MD 6 Training Depot and the CMH, then was SOS in March 1919 and moved to Wolfville, where she continued nursing until retiring in 1927.

38. Campbell, Laura Emily (1883–1956). Born in Glace Bay, Cape Breton, d/o John and Margaret (Cox) Campbell, she was living in Halifax when she shaved four years from her age and joined the CAMCNS in April 1916, naming her sister, Maud Campbell, as NOK. She served in No. 9 CSH, the Westcliffe Canadian Eye and Ear Hospital, No. 6 CGH, No. 12 CGH and No. 16 CGH. She was SOS in August 1919 and was nursing in Saint John, New Brunswick, in 1923. She continued military nursing until retiring to Glace Bay in 1946.

39. Cann, Jessie May (1878–1943). Born in Brenton, Yarmouth County, d/o Jesse (deceased) and Mary Agnes (Crosby) Cann and stepdaughter of Nathaniel Forbes, she was a 1906 graduate of the Worcester City Hospital School of Nursing in Worcester, Massachusetts, and nursed for nine years in hospitals in Massachusetts and New York until joining the American Red Cross in 1917. She served with its Children's Bureau (for refugee children) in Paris, then was sent to Vodena (now Edessa), Greece, to assist in the establishment of a hospital for refugees. She also served at Salonika and on the Italian front in No. 5 American Red Cross Military Hospital at Auteuil, Paris. From December 1918 to March 1919, she nursed in Germany, then with the Red Cross in Vladivostok, caring for refugee children. She returned home in February 1920 and subsequently nursed in a hospital in Greenwich, Connecticut, and in New York. Her brother, Gilbert Franklin Cann, joined the 85th Battalion in October 1915, rose to the rank of lieutenant, and was killed in action in France in January 1918.

40. Canning, Anna Loretta (1890–1951). Born in Springhill, Cumberland County, d/o William and Minnie (Kennedy) Canning, she was living in Halifax and

had CAMC experience when she joined the CAMCNS in November 1916. She served in the DCRC, No. 7 CGH and No. 3 CGH and was SOS in April 1919. In September 1919 she married Harry Scott Chalmers, an electrician from Bathurst, New Brunswick, who had served overseas as a sergeant in the 26th Battalion and was wounded three times. Her brother, Arthur Lorne Canning, served overseas as well in No. 2 Canadian Pioneer Battalion.

41. Chisholm, Christina Elizabeth (1884–1969). Born in St. Andrews, Antigonish County, d/o Donald and Isabel (Chisholm) Chisholm, she studied nursing in the United States and joined the American Ambulance Hospital at Neuilly in August 1914, supported by the US ambassador and wealthy donors. It treated wounded soldiers, ferried them from the front during the First Battle of the Marne in September, aided by volunteer ambulance drivers. She returned to Canada in 1916 and, shaving a year off her date of birth, joined the CAMCNS in April 1916. She served in No. 9 CSH, the Granville Canadian Special Hospital, No. 3 CSH in France, No. 1 CCCS and the Canadian Red Cross Officers Hospital in London, England, until being SOS in August 1919. She later moved to New York but retired to Antigonish.

42. Chisholm, Christine "Christy" Ann. *See* Bowes, Christine "Christy" Ann.

43. Chisholm, Mary Maud Ethel "May" (1883–1966). Born in Halifax, Halifax County, d/o Murdoch and Ada (Clayton) Chisholm, she was a 1915 graduate of the VGH School of Nursing and joined the CAMCNS in October 1915. She served in No. 7 CSH and No. 8 CGH until November 1918 when she resigned and lived with her parents. Her father was a prominent physician in Halifax and professor of clinical surgery at Dalhousie University. He was injured when his home was damaged in the Halifax Explosion in December 1917. Her five brothers, William, Kenneth, George, Alexander, and James also served in the war. William, an engineer, served with the Canadian Engineers. Kenneth, also an engineer, served in the Princess Patricia's Canadian Light Infantry until being wounded and sent home. George, a dentist, served in the 5th Battalion and was killed in action in September 1918. Alexander, a student with the 66th militia regiment, served with the Nova Scotia Railway Construction and Forestry Department, and James, a physician with a year's experience in the Royal Army Medical Corps, transferred into the CEF in September 1916 and served in CHH and its subsidiaries until September 1919.

44. Chisholm, Sarah Catherine (1883–1976). Born in Summerside, Antigonish County, d/o Christopher and Sarah (deceased) (MacDonald) Chisholm, she shaved three years from her date of birth when she joined the CAMCNS in April 1916. She served in No. 9 CSH, No. 2 CSH and No. 10 CSH until being SOS and returning home in July 1919. She moved to Montreal and

was nursing in a private hospital in 1931 but returned home and married William Cameron, a merchant, in 1933.

45. Christie, Frieda Hope (1891–1923). Born in River Hebert, Cumberland County, d/o Edward and Saleah (Neily) Christie of Truro, Colchester County, she attended the Acadia University Seminary (collegiate course). She may have studied nursing in New England because she served for eighteen months in the Harvard Surgical Unit at RAMC No. 22 General Hospital at Étaples. In June 1918 she transferred into the CAMCNS in London and served briefly with No. 10 CSH and No. 16 CGH until being SOS and returning home in February 1919. She died of meningitis in Mexico.

46. Churchill, Sarah Rowena (1878–1964). Born in Yarmouth, Yarmouth County, d/o Joseph and Lydia (Symonds) Churchill, Darling Lake, Yarmouth County, she graduated from St. Joseph's Hospital School of Nursing in Glace Bay and was nursing at the Nova Scotia Sanatorium in Kentville when she joined the CAMCNS in October 1915. She served in No. 7 CSH, No. 16 CGH and on the hospital ship HMAT *Araguaya* until being SOS in Halifax in May 1919, when she resumed nursing at the Kentville sanatorium, retiring in 1949.

47. Clarke, Edith Esther (1894–1976). Born in Annapolis Royal, Annapolis County, d/o Wilbert and Harriet (Hardwick) Clarke, she had three months' CAMC experience when she joined the CAMCNS in July 1918. She served in No. 11 CGH until contracting influenza and returned in April 1919 to Halifax where she served at CHH. In October 1919 she married William Angus Livingstone, a captain in the 25th Battalion who was convalescing at CHH. He subsequently became a lawyer and judge in Annapolis Royal until they moved to New Westminster, British Columbia.

48. Clarke, Katherine Parker (1882–1958). Born in New Glasgow, Pictou County, d/o George and Alice (McKay) Clarke, she joined the CAMCNS in February 1915. She served briefly in No. 2 CGH at Le Tréport and No. 1 CSH at Salonika until contracting malaria and being invalided to England in August 1916. She then served at the DCRC at Taplow, then was transferred to MD 6 in July 1917 and served in CHH and possibly Pine Hill Convalescent Hospital in Halifax. In September 1917 she married John Godson, of New Westminster, BC, who had served overseas in the 7th Battalion, was wounded and convalesced at CHH. When he was transferred to Vancouver for further treatment in September 1917, she remained in Halifax but died in New Glasgow. He never returned and pursued a career in vaudeville and films and died in Culver City, Los Angeles, in 1952.

49. Clements, Eva Beatrice (1885–1972). Born in Liverpool, Queens County, d/o Herbert and Mary (Sholds) Clements, she studied nursing at the McLean Hospital, a psychiatric hospital associated with Harvard University, and at

the Massachusetts General Hospital. She was superintendent of nurses at a Philadelphia hospital when she joined the Harvard Surgical Unit at the RAMC No. 22 General Hospital at Étaples, France. When the US entered the war, she joined the US Army Nurse Service and served until April 1919. She subsequently worked as a public health nurse in Massachusetts until marrying Harry Dary in 1927. They lived in Taunton, Massachusetts, until he died in 1972, when she moved to Chicago.

50. Coates, Dora Evelyn (1888–1929). Born in Dartmouth, Halifax County, d/o Robert and Catherine (MacLean) Coates, she studied nursing at Worcester State Hospital in Worcester, Massachusetts, and took several postgraduate courses in New York hospitals, then returned to Halifax and nursed both there and in Montreal as a Victorian Order of Nurses (VON) sister. She had eight months' CAMC experience when she joined the CAMCNS in July 1918 and served in No. 4 CGH at Basingstoke, England. She was SOS and returned home in July 1919, then moved to Saint John, New Brunswick, where she was in charge of the VON until being appointed superintendent of nurses in a hospital in Cleveland, Ohio, where she died in 1929.

51. Condon, Marguerite (1889–1974). Born in Moncton, New Brunswick, d/o William and Mary Bell (McConnell) Condon, Halifax, she served in the Harvard Surgical Unit at RAMC No. 22 General Hospital at Étaples until transferring into the CAMCNS in London in June 1916. She served in No. 4 CGH, the Granville Canadian Special Hospital and No. 16 CGH. In January 1919 she was posted to Halifax, where she served in CHH and CMC until being SOS in April 1920. In 1922 she married Henry McLeod, a Halifax jeweller. Her brother, Walter Condon, served overseas as well with the No. 1 Overseas Battery, Canadian Siege Artillery.

52. Connell, Monica (1882–1956). Born in New Victoria, Cape Breton, d/o Lawrence and Elizabeth (Carroll) Connell, she was a 1909 graduate of St. Joseph's Hospital School of Nursing in Glace Bay. She shaved three years off her date of birth when she joined the CAMCNS in April 1916 and served in No. 9 CSH. She returned home in March 1919 and served in the Moxham Castle Convalescent Hospital in Sydney until being SOS in May 1919. She was nursing at the Infants' Home in Halifax in 1924–25 but later moved to Montreal and was still nursing there in 1940.

53. Cook, Gertrude Pauline (1876–1957). Born in Halifax, Halifax County, d/o Samuel and Martha (Woodling) Cook, Bridgewater, Lunenburg County, she was a 1904 graduate of the VGH School of Nursing. She was employed with the Department of Immigration at the Halifax Dockyard and had CAMC experience when she shaved eight years from her date of birth and joined the CAMCNS in December 1917. She served in No. 7 CSH until being SOS in

May 1919. She reverted to the CAMC and served in the CMH and CHH until being SOS in December 1919. After the war she returned to Bridgewater and worked as a private nurse until retiring in 1939.

54. Cooke, Elizabeth Ann "Bessie" (1878–1953). Born in Pictou, Pictou County, d/o William and Jessie (Fraser) Cooke, she was a graduate of St. Joseph's Hospital School of Nursing in Glace Bay. She joined the CAMCNS in October 1915, claiming to have been born in 1880, and served in No. 7 CSH and No. 3 CGH. She was mentioned in dispatches and was awarded the Queen Elisabeth Medal (Belgium). In April 1919 she returned to Halifax, reverted to the CAMC and served in CHH and CMH until being SOS in March 1920. She returned to Pictou and continued nursing until 1950.

55. Coolen, Anastasia Muriel (1890–1977). Born at Upper Prospect, Halifax County, d/o Joseph and Ann (Hearn) Coolen, Halifax, and sister of Mary Ellen Coolen (*See* #56), she studied nursing at the Nova Scotia Hospital, a two-year program. That did not qualify her as a trained nurse, but she also had three months' CAMC experience when she shaved six years off her date of birth and joined the CAMCNS in August 1918. She served in CHH and CMH until being SOS in July 1919. Two months later she married Raymond Doherty, a fisherman in Upper Prospect. In about 1949, following his death, she moved to Halifax. Her brother, Patrick Coolen, enlisted in the 40th Battalion but served in the Princess Patricia's Canadian Light Infantry until falling ill and being sent home for treatment at CHH, and was discharged as unfit in January 1918. Her sister, Mary Ellen Coolen, also served as a military nurse.

56. Coolen, Mary Ellen (1873–1947). Born in Upper Prospect, d/o Joseph and Ann (Hearn) Coolen, Halifax, and sister of Anastasia Muriel Coolen (*See* #55), she had CAMC experience when she reduced her date of birth to 1890 and joined the CAMCNS in July 1917, although her service record states elsewhere that she joined in July 1918. She served in CHH and subsidiary hospitals from April to August 1919 when she was SOS. She was still nursing at CHH in 1923 and the Halifax Health Centre No. 1 in 1925. In 1929 she married William Duff Simpson, whose parents had emigrated from England to Bridgewater, then moved to Halifax. He was a bank clerk and had eighteenth months' experience in the 63rd Halifax Rifles but served in the 17th and 85th Battalions, rising to the rank of captain.

57. Corning, Sara (1872–1969). Born in Chegoggin, Yarmouth County, d/o Samuel and Delilah (Churchill) Corning, she trained as a nurse in New Hampshire and served in the Halifax Explosion recovery, then joined the American Red Cross and was assigned to Near East Relief, a charitable foundation that assisted the displaced populations of the Balkans and

the Middle East. She established an orphanage in Armenia and worked in refugee camps, then was stationed at Smyrna (now Izmir) where she rescued some five thousand Armenian children and established an orphanage on the Greek island of Syros. Greece's King George II awarded her the Silver Cross Medal of the Order of the Saviour. She later returned to Turkey to work in a residential training school and adopted five children, then retired to Chegoggin. In September 2012 the Canadian Armenian community established the Sara Corning Centre for Genocide Education to promote human rights education and encourage Canadian students to engage in civic life, advocate for their own rights and those of others, and be aware of the consequences of discrimination.[193]

58. Cornwell, Bertha Jennie (1881–1967). Born in Little River, Kings County, d/o Henry and Alice (deceased) (Stanton) Cornwell and stepdaughter of Jennie (Clark) Cornwell, she studied nursing at the Massachusetts General Hospital's School of Nursing in Boston until joining the US Army Nurse Corps. She was awarded the French Croix de Guerre for her service at Field Hospital No. 12 through twelve hours of shelling in October 1918. After the war she returned to the United States and in 1920 was superintendent of nurses in a hospital in Geneva, New York, and in several other hospitals in the eastern United States, including New London, Connecticut, in 1935 and Wernersville State Hospital, South Heidelberg, Pennsylvania, in 1940. By 1950 she had retired and lived in Winter Park, Pinellas, Florida, and died in St. Petersburg, Florida. Her brother, Harry Allen Cornwall, enlisted in the 40th Battalion in 1915 but served with the Canadian Army Pay Corps in England.

59. Cray, Bertha Geraldine (1890–1975). Born in Dartmouth, Halifax County, d/o William and Bertha (Shute) Cray. Her father had been a Royal Hospital Chelsea Pensioner in England for several years when he and his family emigrated to Dartmouth. When he died in 1894, her mother, who worked as a teacher, married Charles Murray, a railway worker in Saint John, New Brunswick, who also died. Bertha, the daughter, appears to have trained in nursing in Massachusetts because she served with the Harvard Surgical Unit at RAMC No. 22 General Hospital at Étaples in France. In June 1916 she transferred into the CAMCNS in London and served in No. 4 CSH at Salonika until contracting malaria and returning to England. She also served on the *Llandovery Castle* hospital ship and in No. 12 CGH until being SOS in July 1919. In 1923 she married Robert Goulding Simpson, a farmer whose family had emigrated from England and settled at Innisfree, Alberta. He enlisted in the 51st Battalion in Edmonton in 1915 but served in the 49th Battalion in France, until being plagued with influenza, typhoid

fever and other health issues and was SOS in May 1919.[194] She died in 1975, followed by her husband in 1977.

60. Crockett, Edith. *See* Anderson, Edith.
61. Cruikshank, Adam Joseph (1890–1936). Born in Sheet Harbour, Halifax County, s/o Martin and Bridget (Redmond) Cruikshank and husband of Bertha (Henneberry) Cruikshank, he was a 1912 graduate of the VGH School of Nursing and was nursing in the Halifax Infirmary when he joined the CAMCNS in June 1917 but as an orderly. He served in the MD 6 Training Depot until January 1918, when he was SOS as "medically unfit" and died of epilepsy in the Halifax City Home (formerly named the City Poor Asylum).
62. Cumming, Isabel Katherine (1881–1921). Born in Melrose, Pictou County, d/o Rev. Robert and Corinna (Grant) Cumming, Westville, Pictou County, she joined the CAMCNS in London in May 1915. She served in No. 3 CSH at Rouen and No. 1 CGH at Étaples until being diagnosed with pulmonary tuberculosis in December 1915 in London. She was sent home and was treated in the Nova Scotia Sanatorium until dying at home in New Glasgow.
63. Currie, Alice Margaret (1890–1951). Born in Pictou, Pictou County, d/o William and Margaret (Robertson Talbot) Currie, she was a 1914 graduate of the VGH School of Nursing and had sixteen months' CAMC militia experience when she joined the CAMCNS in July 1918. She served in No. 11 CGH and No. 15 CGH until being SOS in October 1919. She subsequently moved to Vancouver and presumably nursed in the Vancouver General Hospital because in 1938 she married George Samuel Haddon, its secretary and "a prominent Vancouver figure." Their home in Burnaby, built in 1923 by Haddon and his first wife (deceased), is a heritage property considered "a significant example of the romantic period revival styles that were popular during the period between the two World Wars."[195]
64. Davidson, Jessie Ann (1885–1958). Born in Banffshire, Scotland, d/o James and Jessie (Davidson) Davidson, Halifax, she was a 1910 graduate of the VGH School of Nursing and was operating room supervisor in the VGH when she joined the CAMCNS in October 1915. She served in No. 7 CSH, RAMC No. 2 Stationary Hospital and No. 3 CGH until being SOS in March 1918. She returned to Halifax and served in CHH and subsidiaries until January 1920 when she married Dr. John Robert Mitchell Colley, a 1911 graduate of the Dalhousie Medical School, who was born in River John, Pictou County. He then pursued postgraduate studies in London but then returned to Canada and served in the Royal Canadian Navy in the war. They subsequently returned to London, England, until 1928 when he was appointed assistant medical officer for the Confederation Life Insurance Company in Toronto, then chief medical officer in 1937, retiring in 1954. He is listed on the River John War Memorial as Major J. R. M. Colley.

65. Davies, Edith Maria (1891–?). Born in Halifax, Halifax County, d/o John and Florence Davies, who had emigrated in 1909 from Wales to Nova Scotia, where her father was sergeant major of the 63rd Halifax Rifles Regiment. She studied nursing in Newton Hospital in Newton, Massachusetts, then moved to Montreal where she nursed in the Drummond Military Convalescent Hospital until joining the CAMCNS in May 1917, naming her father as NOK. She served in CHH and subsidiaries in Halifax but contracted pneumonia and influenza and was SOS in June 1919. She then returned to Montreal where, according to the 1921 Canadian census, she had married James Daives, a wheelwright from Poland, who worked in a railway shop. She was no longer nursing because they had two sons. He died before 1931, and that year's census stated that the "wife, son, [and] daughter [were] working without regular wages."[196]
66. Davies, Margaret Emily (1889–1930). Born in Widnes, Lancashire, England, d/o Edwin and Margaret (Hughes) Davies, Springhill, Cumberland County, she was nursing in Saint John, New Brunswick, when she joined the CAMCNS in Halifax in April 1917. She served in No. 11 CGH at Shorncliffe and No. 12 CGH at Bramshott Camp until returning to Halifax in September 1919 for health reasons and was SOS in December 1919. She returned to Springhill and in 1920 married Harold Fraser, a Springhill tailor who had served as a sergeant in the 46th Battalion, was wounded, and was awarded the Meritorious Service Medal. After the war he was a customs officer until dying in 1933 of a gunshot that may or may not have been accidental..
67. Dawson, Isabell Helen (1889–1955). Born in Boston, Massachusetts, d/o Chipman and Joanne "Jane" (Walsh) Dawson. The family was living in Little Harbour, Pictou County, in 1891. She studied nursing in Hudson County, New Jersey, and joined the CAMCNS in April 1916. She served in No. 9 CSH, the Granville Canadian Special Hospital, No. 6 CGH and No. 12 CGH until being SOS in July 1919. She married Angus MacArthur, a businessman in New Glasgow, Pictou County, who had joined the 64th Battalion but served overseas in the 42nd Battalion.
68. Dempsey, Mary Catharine (1882–1962). Born in Halifax, Halifax County, d/o John (deceased) and Janet (Fitzgerald) Dempsey, she had CAMC experience when she joined the CAMCNS in December 1916. She served in No. 2 CGH and No. 15 CGH until being returned to Halifax in February 1918. She reverted to the CAMC and was posted to CMH and CHH. She was demobilized in April 1920 and later lived in Chatham, New Brunswick.
69. Desmond, Mary Ann (1888[197]–1978). Born in Granton, Pictou County, d/o Daniel and Mary (McKenna) Desmond, she may have graduated from St. Joseph's Hospital because she was working as a private nurse in Glace Bay in 1911 for the family of William Carroll, a lawyer and the member of

parliament for Cape Breton South from 1911 to 1917, who was defeated in the 1917 conscription election even though he had joined the 185th Battalion.[198] She joined the CAMCNS in August 1918 and served at CHH and subsidiaries until being SOS in March 1920. She moved to Vancouver in 1921, then to Seattle, Washington, in 1926 and became an American citizen but appears to have died in Montreal in 1978. Her brother, Edward Desmond, enlisted in the 193rd Battalion in 1916 but served in the 42nd Battalion, was seriously wounded, and was invalided home in May 1918.

70. DeWolfe, Anna Clarke Crerar (1893–1977). Born in Halifax, Halifax County, d/o Frederick Turner and Ann Clarke (Crerar) (deceased) DeWolfe and stepdaughter of Edith (Shafner) DeWolfe, she had fourteen months' CAMC experience when she joined the CAMCNS in February 1918. She served in England in No. 14 CGH, No. 9 CGH and No. 16 CGH until being SOS in August 1919. In 1922 she married Edward Davison, a businessman from Detroit and Ypsilanti, Michigan, who died in 1948. Her father, who had two years' experience with the Princess Louise Fusiliers, served in MD 6 as No. 1 Canadian Garrison Artillery's recruiting officer and also commanded the Depot Unit of Supply and its hospital section but proved not to be physically or emotionally suitable, so he was SOS in February 1919 and joined his wife, Edith, who had moved to Vancouver.

71. Dodd, Frances Mary (1884–1972). Born in Sydney, Cape Breton, d/o Dr. Marcus and Sarah (Rigby) Dodd, Bridgeport, Cape Breton, she may have studied nursing at St. Joseph's Hospital in Glace Bay or in the United States. In 1916 she travelled to England and joined the QAIMNS, returning home in October 1918. She married Allan Ridgway, a British war veteran who had served in the 12th Manchester Battalion and was awarded the Military Medal at Neuvilly during the Somme offensive. Perhaps because they had met during the war, he emigrated in 1920 to Cape Breton, where he was employed for forty years by the Metropolitan Life Insurance Company as manager of the North Sydney branch and later as accountant in the Sydney office.

72. Doull, Jessie Cameron (1880–1936). Born in New Glasgow, Pictou County, d/o James Forbes and Christina "Christy" (McLellan) Doull (deceased) and stepdaughter of Irene (Chisholm) Doull, she was living in Halifax and had three months' CAMC militia experience when she shaved four years off her date of birth and joined the CEF in April 1918. She served at CHH and subsidiaries until being SOS because of health issues in April 1919. She subsequently moved to Winnipeg. Her brother, James Angus Doull, a physician, served in the RAMC and received the Military Cross and the Croix de Guerre in recognition of his services.

73. Doyle, Elizabeth Cecilia (1874–1952). Born in Dartmouth, Halifax County, d/o Daniel and Bridget (Stevens) Brennan (both deceased), and widow of Dr. Joseph Doyle, a physician at the VGH who had died in 1911, she listed her brother, Daniel Brennan, as NOK. She was an 1898 graduate of the VGH School of Nursing and was one of the eleven nurses who founded the Graduate Nurses' Association of Nova Scotia (GNANS) in 1909. She had four years' CAMC experience and was matron of the CMH when she joined the CAMCNS in June 1918. She initially worked as a private nurse, served in No. 3 CGH, No. 16 CGH and No. 15 CGH until returning in June 1919 to Halifax, where she served at CHH and CMH until being demobilized in April 1920. That same year she married Dr. E. V. Hogan, professor of surgery at Dalhousie University's Medical School, who had succeeded Dr. John Stewart in command of No. 7 CSH and was wounded when it was bombed in May 1918. He received the Commander of the Order of the British Empire (CBE) for his services. She subsequently worked in public health and child welfare and was awarded posthumously the Centennial Award of Distinction by the College of Registered Nurses.[199]
74. Drew, Margaret Currie (1885–1959). Born in Liverpool, Queens County, d/o Lemuel and Amelia (Sprague) Drew, she was a 1909 graduate of the Women's Charity Club Hospital in Boston. She joined the CAMCNS in February 1915, shaving a year off her date of birth, and served in No. 2 CGH, No. 1 CCCS, No. 12 CGH and No. 9 CGH when it was at Kinmel Park. She returned home in June 1919 and served at CHH until 1920 when she was demobilized. She resumed nursing in Liverpool and was still working in 1931.
75. Drummond, Albert William (1887–1961). Born in Scotland, husband of Lillian (Jones) Drummond, he and his family moved to Halifax via New York. When he joined the CAMC in December 1916, he claimed to be a nurse, but he was not hospital trained and later described himself as a masseur. He served at the Cooden Military Camp at Bexhill, England, and No. 15 Field Ambulance in England until June 1918 when he served in No. 14 Canadian Field Ambulance in France. He returned home in August 1919. The family moved to Kenosha, Wisconsin, where his parents lived, but then moved to Guelph, Ontario, and then Seattle, Washington. He published two small books of poetry, *Fat-i-gue* (1916) and *Rhymes of a Hut-Dweller* (1918) and a history of Guelph, entitled *Guelph: The Royal City* (1924).
76. Duff, Margaret Elizabeth Ann "Lida" (1879–1964). Born in Westville, Pictou County, d/o John (deceased) and Elizabeth (Sutherland) Duff, Sydney, Cape Breton, she was a 1907 graduate of the VGH School of Nursing and had CAMC experience when she shaved four years from her date of birth and joined the CAMCNS in Montreal in August 1916. She was sent in Sep-

tember 1916 to England, where she was temporarily attached to No. 2 New Zealand General Hospital, Granville Canadian Special Hospital, and No. 5 CGH and No. 4 CGH at Salonika. In October 1916 she returned to England and served in the Canadian Red Cross Officers Hospital at Bushy Park, London. She somehow met James Percy McNaughton, a Montreal-based sales manager of the Dominion Iron and Steel Company, who was there on business, and they married and returned home in February 1918.[200] When he died suddenly in 1920, she moved to Smiths Cove, Digby County, and died there but was buried in Westville.

77. Dunbar, Lilian Cameron (1873–1935). Born in Montreal, Quebec, d/o William and Elizabeth (Hickman) Renshaw and wife of Dr. William Dunbar, Truro, Colchester County, she was a graduate of the RVH School of Nursing and had six months' CAMC experience when she shaved ten years off her date of birth and joined the CAMCNS in Halifax in October 1918. She served in CHH and CMH until being SOS in December 1919. William served as mayor of Truro from about 1917 to 1928, and when the Halifax Explosion took place, "arranged for a special train carrying doctors—including himself—nurses, firefighters and equipment to go to Halifax." It arrived shortly after noon and "around 3:30 P.M. the first trainload of injured arrived in Truro, where emergency medical centres had been set up."[201] He was active in the Nova Scotia Medical Society and served as president in 1931. Her death certificate states that she had been seriously ill since 1920.

78. Dunlap, Laura Alice (1882–1972). Born in Ellershouse, Hants County, d/o Tom Gibbs and Emma (Barnaby) Dunlap, Halifax, she had fifteen months' CAMC experience when she joined the CAMCNS in June 1918. She served in England at No. 5 CGH and No. 16 CGH and was SOS in September 1919. She was living in Halifax from 1921 to 1927, then moved to California and was living in Pasadena in 1940. She became a US citizen in 1951 and died in nearby Altadena.

79. Duthie, Edna Craig (1890–1976). Born in Salmon River, Colchester County, d/o James and Helen (Ferguson) Duthie, New Glasgow, Pictou County, she had CAMC experience when she joined the CEF in January 1917. She served in the Kitchener Military Hospital (redesignated No. 10 CGH in September 1917), No. 6 CGH, No. 2 CGH and No. 16 CGH, and was awarded the Médaille d'honneur des Epidemies en Bronze by the French government. In May 1919 she was transferred to Halifax where she served at CHH until being SOS in August 1919. She was nursing in the Municipal Hospital in Winnipeg in 1921 but returned to New Glasgow by 1957. Her brother, Stewart Muir Duthie, served overseas with the 4th Divisional Ammunition Column and was killed in action in August 1918.

80. Eaton, Evangeline "May" (1892–1988). Born in Canard, Kings County, d/o Everard (deceased) and Evangeline (North) Eaton, and a cousin of Sir Frederick Borden, she attended the Acadia University Seminary (collegiate course). Like many young people from Canard, she moved to Roxbury, Massachusetts, in 1911 or 1912 to study nursing. She remained there until the war broke out when she joined the Harvard Surgical Unit, likely serving in the RAMC No. 22 General Hospital at Étaples. After the war she continued nursing in the United States, settling in Ukiah, Mendocino, California, where she nursed in the nearby Mendocino State Hospital for Insane, became a citizen in 1965, and died there but was buried in Canard.[202]
81. Edgecombe, Lillian Grace (1877–1949). Born in Dartmouth, Halifax County, d/o Richard (deceased) and Annie (Shiers) Edgecombe, she studied nursing in Boston and served for eleven months with the Harvard Surgical Unit in the RAMC No. 22 General Hospital at Étaples before shaving two years off her date of birth and joining the CAMCNS in London in June 1916. She served with No. 1 CSH, No. 4 CGH at Salonika, the CAMC Depot at Shorncliffe, the Canadian Convalescent Hospital at Bearwood Park, No. 3 CSH, No. 8 CSH and the King's Canadian Red Cross Hospital at Bushy Park before being SOS in June 1919. In 1925 she married John Sampson Misener, originally from Boston but living in Dartmouth, whose first wife (Alice Burchell) had died in 1919. Lillian described herself in the marriage register as a housewife. Her brother, Harold Edgecombe, who had moved to Grouard, Alberta, was conscripted in November 1917, served in the 50th Battalion, and was wounded in October 1918.
82. Ellis, Helena Margaret (1894–1959). Born in Shubenacadie, Colchester County, d/o Morton and Mary (Guild) Ellis, she was a graduate of the Danvers State Hospital School of Nursing in Danvers, Massachusetts. She was nursing in Englewood, New Jersey, when she returned home and joined No. 9 CSH in April 1916, shaving eight years off her date of birth. She also served in No. 12 CGH, No. 6 CGH, No. 2 CGH, No. 7 CGH, No. 4 CCCS, No. 16 CGH and the Granville Canadian Special Hospital. She was SOS in August 1919 and returned to Halifax. After unsuccessfully seeking a position in the postwar Canadian Army Nursing Corps, she nursed in White Plains, New York; Edmonton, Alberta, and Winnipeg, Manitoba, where she married Otto Koch, a farmer. Her brother, Alonzo Ellis, was conscripted in June 1918 and served with the Nova Scotia Regiment Depot Battalion in Halifax.
83. Ellis, Marion Dean (1885–1967). Born in Upper Stewiacke, Colchester County, d/o Willard and Annie (Dean) Ellis, Truro, Colchester County, she studied nursing in Boston and served for nine months with the Harvard Surgical Unit at RAMC No. 22 General Hospital at Étaples. In September 1917 she

transferred into the CAMCNS in London and served in No. 10 CGH, No. 7 CGH and No. 15 CGH and was SOS in July 1919. She returned home but later lived in Cleveland, Ohio. Her brother, Hugh Ellis, joined the CEF and served in the 14th Brigade, Canada Field Artillery.

84. Etherington, Ethel Florence Bingay (1880–1964). Born in Shelburne, Shelburne County, d/o Robert and Catherine (Bingay) Etherington, she had ten months' experience with the Harvard Surgical Unit at RAMC No. 22 General Hospital at Étaples when she transferred into the CAMCNS in London in April 1916. She served in No. 2 CGH and No. 2 CSH but developed health issues and returned to Halifax in March 1919, serving in CHH until being demobilized in January 1920. In 1925 she married Harold Draper, who had served overseas in the 26th Battalion but was sent home in 1917 because of health issues requiring surgery and convalesced at CHH. They lived in Shelburne until he died in 1933. She subsequently moved to Yarmouth, retiring from nursing in 1945.

85. Ferguson, Lydia Reata (1881–1957). Born in Yarmouth, Yarmouth County, d/o Richard and Lydia (Dennis) Ferguson, she was nursing in the United States by 1911 and joined the Harvard Surgical Unit at RAMC No. 22 General Hospital at Étaples. She also served in Northwestern University Base Hospital No. 12, the second US hospital unit to go to France, where it took over the RAMC No. 18 Hospital at Camiers. In October 1918 she received a citation for remaining on duty when the hospital was shelled for twelve hours. She subsequently served with the American Red Cross Palestine Commission in Palestine, Syria and Egypt, then returned to Yarmouth in July 1919 and married William Kirk, a local merchant.[203]

86. Fife, Lillian Jessie (1889–1981). Born in Millville, Cape Breton, d/o Robert and Mary (Morrison) Fife, she was a 1915 graduate of the VGH School of Nursing and had sixteen months' experience in the CAMC when she joined the CAMCNS in April 1918. She served in No. 4 CGH, No. 14 CGH, No. 9 CGH and No. 15 CGH until being SOS in July 1919. She nursed with the VON in Sydney, retiring in the 1950s.

87. Fitzgerald, Lillian Mary (1889–1952). Born at Portuguese Cove, Halifax County, d/o James (deceased) and Margaret (O'Neill) Fitzgerald, Halifax, she was a 1914 graduate of the VGH School of Nursing and joined the CAMCNS in October 1915. She served in No. 7 CSH, RAMC No. 2 Stationary Hospital at Abbeville, and was briefly acting matron in No. 4 CGH, until being SOS in April 1919 and returning to Halifax. She served at CHH until being discharged in January 1920 but continued working there until a month before her death. Her brother, James Fitzgerald, joined the 40th Battalion but was transferred into the 25th Battalion, was promoted to lieutenant, was wounded in 1918 and was awarded the Military Cross.

88. Follette, Minnie Asenath (1884–1918). Born in Port Greville, Cumberland County, d/o Oscar and Lydia (Hatfield) Follette, Ward's Brook, Cumberland County, she was a 1909 graduate of the VGH School of Nursing. She joined the CAMC in November 1911 and the CAMCNS in September 1914 and went overseas with the first CEF contingent. She served in No. 1 CCCS and No. 2 CGH until April 1916, when she was declared unfit for service for two months because of nervous strain, then was transferred to No. 9 CSH and No. 16 CGH. That was why Matron-in-Chief Macdonald posted her to transport service on the *Llandovery Castle* hospital ship in June 1918, a policy that she had developed for nurses who needed a break from the stress of their work and a visit with their families. Much to Macdonald's horror, Follette was one of the fourteen nurses who died when it was torpedoed on June 27, 1918.

M.A. Follette, drowned by the torpedoeing of H.M. Hospital Ship
Llandovery Castle June 27 1918.

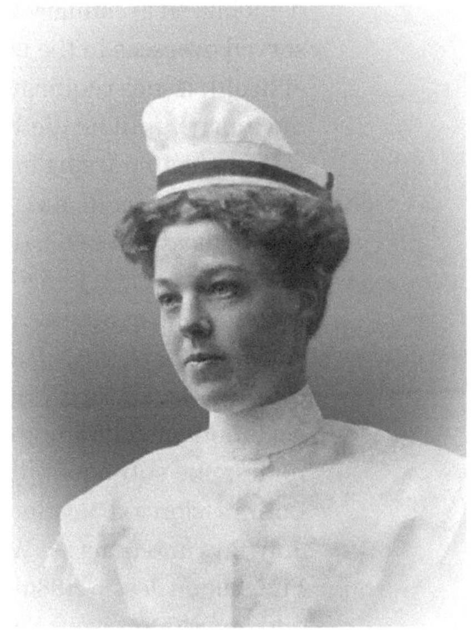

Minnie Follette. [VICTORIA GENERAL HOSPITAL SCHOOL OF NURSING ARCHIVES]

89. Fox, Dorothy Gayton (1889–1952). Born in Pubnico, Yarmouth County, d/o Dr. Charles and Deidama "Annie" (Gayton) (deceased) Fox, she studied nursing at the Malden Hospital School of Nursing in Malden, Massachusetts, and joined the US Army Nurse Corps in Canton, Massachusetts, in December 1917. After training at the base hospital at Camp Sevier, South Carolina, she was sent overseas and served as a surgical nurse in French hospitals: No. 24 Base Hospital at Limoges, No. 1 Evacuation Hospital at Argonne Forest, Sebastopol Barracks at Toul, No. 37 Evacuation Hospital, Camp Hospital No. 8 at Montigny-le-Roi, and the Hospital Centre at Vannes. She was SOS in May 1919, received the US Victory Medal in 1920, and moved to Los Angeles, where she became an American citizen and married Ray Daniel. They lived in Berkeley in the 1930s. Her brother, Lyle Fox, enlisted in Nova Scotia's 40th Battalion in 1915 and rose to the rank of lieutenant in the 26th Battalion, was wounded and was awarded the Distinguished Conduct Medal and the Military Medal. Her sister, Annie Gayton Fox, also joined the US Army Nurse Corps and served in the First World War and through the 1920s and 1930s was the chief nurse at Hickam Field in Hawaii when Japan attacked

Pearl Harbor in December 1941. She was the first US service woman to be awarded the Purple Heart for "performance of duty and meritorious acts of extraordinary fidelity,"[204] which included working as an anaesthetist in the station hospital. She subsequently rose to the rank of major, retiring in 1945 in San Diego, California.

90. Fraser, Annie Margaret (1892–1975). Born in Iron Rock, Pictou County, d/o Charles and Jane (MacDonald) Fraser, she was a 1914 graduate of the VGH School of Nursing. She was nursing in Halifax and had sixteen months' CAMC experience when she joined the CAMCNS in May 1917. She served in No. 9 CSH, No. 12 CGH, and No. 4 CGH until returning home in June 1919 and being posted to CHH. She was demobilized in January 1920 and spent two years in charge of a private clinic in Yarmouth and did private-duty nursing in Halifax, including sixteen years with the family of James Tory, a prominent businessman who was also the Liberal MLA for Guysborough County from 1911 to 1925, minister without portfolio from 1921 to 1925, and lieutenant governor from 1925 to 1930. She was awarded the King George V Silver Jubilee Medal in 1935 and in 1961 was made a life member of the VGH School of Nursing Alumnae Association.

91. Fraser, Edith Lilian Morrow[205] (1886–1939). Born in Halifax, Halifax County, d/o James and Edith (Neal) Fraser (both deceased), she lived in Montclair, New Jersey, with her sister, Muriel Fraser, while she studied nursing at St. Luke's Hospital in New York City. She had CAMC militia experience in Montreal when she joined the CAMCNS in May 1917, naming Muriel as NOK. She served in the Canadian Red Cross Officers Hospital in London, the DCRC, No. 15 CGH and No. 3 CGH, and was awarded the Royal Red Cross 2nd Class. She was SOS at Halifax in May 1919 and was nursing in Arichat in 1935 and may have died there in 1939.[206]

92. Fraser, Elda Jean (1883–1958). Born in Alma, Pictou County, d/o Archibald and Elizabeth (Huggan) (deceased) Fraser, she studied nursing and nursed in Boston from 1905 to 1910, until her mother died in 1912, and she returned home. She had CAMC experience and joined the CAMCNS in March 1917. She served in No. 9 CGH until being transferred to Halifax in June 1918 because of health issues. Somehow, she met Robert Blair Campbell, a banker from Richmond, Virginia, and married him in Alma in 1922. They lived in Richmond, where she died. Her brother, (George) Alvin Fraser, joined the 193rd Battalion but served in the 85th Battalion and was wounded.

93. Fraser, Florence Amelia (1891–1957). Born in Flatlands, Restigouche County, New Brunswick, d/o James and Emma (Gettings) Fraser, she was living in Halifax and her family joined her, perhaps because she was already

there. She served at CHH and joined the CAMC, claiming to be a year older than she was, when she joined the CAMCNS in July 1918. After being SOS in September 1919, she continued nursing in Halifax and was at the Dalhousie Public Health Clinic in 1924–25. Later she moved to Amherst, where she nursed and died in 1956, although her tombstone claims that she died in 1957.[207]

94. Fraser, Florence Matilda (1880–1963). Born in Charlottetown, PEI, d/o Gordon and Ann (Stewart) Fraser, New Glasgow, Pictou County, she was a 1908 graduate of the VGH School of Nursing. She was nursing at Harbourview Hospital in Sydney Mines when she joined No. 7 CSH in December 1915. She served in England and France until being SOS in November 1917 and returning to Halifax, where she served in the CMH until being demobilized in January 1920. She moved to New York City in 1923 but was living in Glace Bay, Cape Breton, in 1924–25, then later moved to Montreal and died there.[208]

95. Fraser, Frances Margaret (1872–1948). Born in Pictou, Pictou County, d/o Frederick Wyatt and Sarah Jane (Dickson) Fraser (both deceased), she had sixteen months' CAMC experience when she joined the CAMCNS in July 1918. She served at the MD 6 Training Depot and CHH from January to July 1919. In 1923 she was nursing at No. 2 Health Centre in Dartmouth,[209] then the Dalhousie Public Health Clinic in 1924–25 but later moved to Montreal and died there.[210]

96. Fraser, Lavinia Flora (1877–1961). Born in Bermuda, she appears to have moved to Nova Scotia with her parents, Rose (deceased) and Mary (Masters) Fraser, in 1898, settling on a farm at Truro, Colchester County. In 1901 she moved to Esquimalt, BC, where she was employed as a governess but subsequently returned to her family in Halifax, perhaps when her father died in 1905. She was a 1908 graduate of the VGH School of Nursing and had three years' CAMC experience at CMH when she joined the CAMCNS in September 1918 despite being over age. She served in the MD 6 Training Depot and No. 16 CGH in England until being SOS in July 1919. She continued nursing in Halifax until at least 1949. Her brother Lewis Hayes Fraser, a Halifax physician with nine years' CAMC experience, served overseas as a captain in the CAMC, was wounded in October 1918, and received the Military Cross. Another brother, Leveson Gower Fraser, was conscripted in October 1917 and served in No. 10 Halifax Siege Battery. In November 1919 he married Kathleen Martina Hallisey, a Nova Scotian nurse who had served briefly in No. 15 CGH but was SOS in June 1919. *See* Hallisey, Kathleen Martina.

97. Fraser, Margaret Anna (1891–1981). Born in Antigonish, Antigonish County, d/o Donald and Mary (Macdonald) Fraser, Marydale, Antigonish County, she had CAMC experience when she joined the CAMCNS in Halifax in January 1917. She served with No. 2 CGH, No. 6 CGH and the Forestry Corps Hospital at Lajoux, going to England in April 1919 and serving in No. 14 CGH and No. 16 CGH. She returned to Halifax and was SOS in August 1919, then moved to New York City, where she met James Paul O'Brien, a stationary clerk. They married in 1927 and in 1940 moved to Teaneck, New Jersey. It is not known if she continued nursing, but he died in 1969, and she died in 1981.[211]

98. Fraser, Margaret Marjory "Pearl" (1885–1918). Born in New Glasgow, Pictou County, d/o Duncan (deceased) and Bessie (Graham) Fraser and a cousin of Harriet Graham (*See* #110), she was a 1909 graduate of the Lady Stanley Institute for Trained Nurses in Ottawa (later the Ottawa Civic Hospital School of Nursing) and had served as head nurse at Vancouver General Hospital but moved to Moose Jaw, Saskatchewan, because her sister and mother lived there. In September 1914 she joined No. 1 CGH in Quebec City but transferred into No. 2 CSH in November, then No. 2 CCCS, which operated a British hospital at Aire-sur-la-Lys, near Béthune, until returning to England in May 1917 and being posted to HMHS *Letitia*. She then was transferred to King's Canadian Red Cross Special Hospital at Bushy Park as "nurse in charge" but after a few months was given leave to Canada. On her return she was assigned to the HMHS *Araguaya*, and then as acting matron on HMHS *Llandovery Castle*, and was one of the fourteen nurses who died when it was torpedoed on June 27, 1918. Her father was a prominent lawyer, mayor, member of parliament from 1891 to 1904, a judge in the Nova Scotia Supreme Court, and lieutenant governor from 1906 until his death in 1910. Her brother James Laurier Fraser died in March 1918 while serving as a lieutenant with the 16th Battalion. Another brother, Alistair Fraser, joined the 17th Battalion in 1914 but served in the 15th as a captain, then major, was wounded and awarded

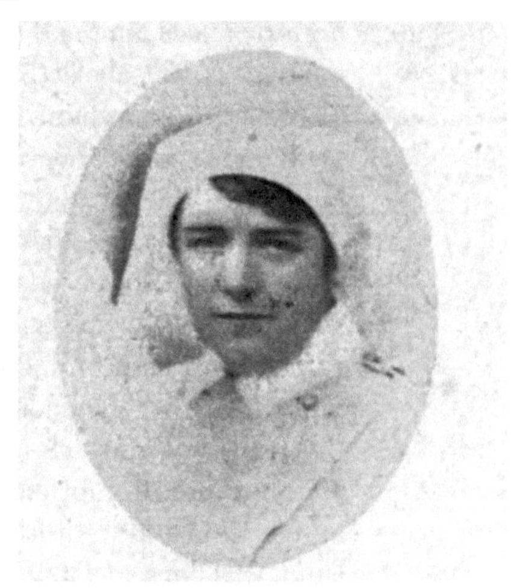

Matron Margaret Fraser. [COMMONWEALTH WAR GRAVES COMMISSION]

the Military Cross following the battle at Vimy Ridge. He subsequently was appointed aide-de-camp to General Arthur Currie but resigned after the deaths of his brother and sister and was assigned administrative duties with MD 12 (Regina). He later served as lieutenant governor of Nova Scotia from 1952 to 1958.

99. Frazee, Gertrude (1884–1980). Born in Dartmouth, Halifax County, d/o John and Ermina (Nowlan) Frazee, she was nursing in Halifax and had CAMC experience when she joined the CAMCNS in February 1917, naming her sister, Laura (Frazee) Hart, as NOK. She served in the Kitchener Military Hospital (redesignated No. 10 CGH in September 1917) in Brighton, England, No. 14 CGH, No. 1 CSH, Granville Canadian Special Hospital and No. 4 CGH until being SOS in August 1919. She enrolled in the first public health nursing diploma course at the University of British Columbia in 1920 and worked in Vancouver, much of the time with her brother Frederick, who was a chiropractor in Richmond. She lived with another brother, Costello Weston Frazee, a banker, and his family. She never married, allegedly because her fiancé died in the sinking of the *Titanic* in 1912. She died in Shaughnessy Military Hospital and donated her remains to the University of British Columbia for research.[212]

100. Frew, Frances Maitland (1879–1965). Born in St. John's, Newfoundland, d/o Henry and Isabella (Blackwood) Blair, and wife of William Syme Frew (deceased), a merchant,[213] she reduced her age by two years when she took a one-month course for officers at the CAMC Divisional School of Military Instruction in Quebec City, then joined the CAMCNS at Valcartier. She went overseas with the first contingent of nurses on the *Franconia* in October 1914 and served in No. 1 CGH at Étaples, No. 1 CCCS at Fort Gassion and No. 2 CCS at Bailleul, where she met Major John Garnet Wolseley Hunt, an oculist from London, Ontario, who had two years' experience in the CAMC when he joined No. 1 CGH at Valcartier in September 1914, the same unit in which Frew served. She became pregnant in July 1916 and they married in October 1916. She was SOS as "permanently unfit" at that time and went to London, Ontario, where their son, John Blair Hunt, was born in January 1917. After a visit home, her husband, now a major, returned overseas and was appointed officer commanding the Anglo-Russian Hospital in Petrograd, Russia, and took part in the retreat from Galicia to Russia and was awarded the Russian Cross of St. Vladimir and discharged in 1918. Their son joined the army in 1940, went overseas with the Princess Patricia's Canadian Light Infantry in 1942, and was killed at Ortona, Italy, in December 1943.

101. Fulton, Mary Sophia (1889–1980). Born in Stewiacke, Colchester County, d/o Rupert and Mary (Dunlap) Fulton, she remained in Nova Scotia studying nursing when her parents moved to Vernon, North Okanagan, British Columbia, in 1910. She later joined them until October 1914, when she joined the CAMCNS in Vancouver. She was sent to England in May 1915, just in time to be sent to Lemnos with No. 3 CSH. She also served in the Moore Barracks Hospital, No. 1 CCCS, No. 2 CGH, No. 6 CGH, No. 11 CGH and the CAMC Casualty Company at Shorncliffe. In March 1917 she served on a hospital ship taking convalescent soldiers back to Canada, which was stopped by a German submarine and searched by its officers, who Fulton told family and friends "were very courteous to the nurses while they searched the ship." She was SOS in February 1919 and nursed in Vancouver, where she married John Archibald Street, an American who had graduated from the McGill University medical school in 1919. They moved to Vernon, BC, and died there.[214] Its museum claims that the Fulton Secondary School in the community is named after Mary's brother, Chester Clarence Fulton, who served in Nova Scotia's 85th Battalion, but the school is actually named after Clarence Fulton, a former principal of several Vernon schools.[215]

102. Gass, Clare (1887–1968). Born in Shubenacadie, Hants County, d/o Robert and Nerissa (Miller) Gass, she was the oldest of ten children and the only girl. She was a 1912 graduate of the MGH School of Nursing and worked as a private duty nurse in Montreal until joining No. 3 CGH in April 1915. She also served in No. 2 CCCS until being sent home in December 1918, after which she served on hospital ships. Happily, she kept a diary that was published in 2000 by Susan Mann as *The War Diary of Clare Gass, 1915–1918* (McGill-Queen's University Press, 2000). After being demobilized in 1919, she returned to Montreal and left nursing to study social work at McGill University and medical social work at Simmons College in Boston, then became head of MGH's Department of Social Work in the Western Division until retiring to Shubenacadie. Three of her brothers served in the war. Gerald enlisted in the

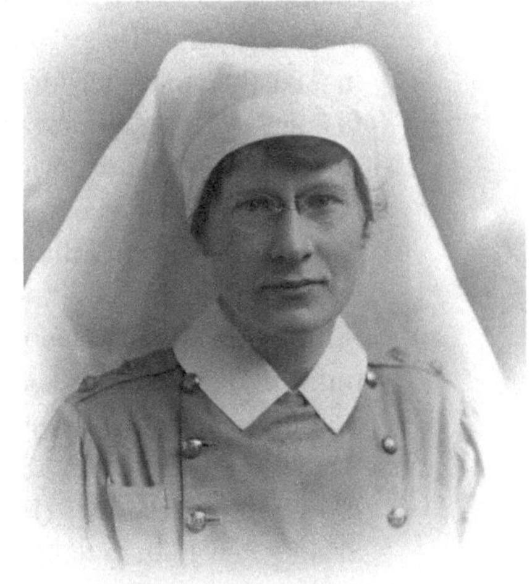

Clare Gass. [PARKS CANADA]

3rd Division Signal Company, Cyril served in the 25th Battalion and was wounded, and Blanchard served in the 85th Battalion and was killed at the age of nineteen at Vimy Ridge.

103. Gates, Sarah Gladys (1888–1952). Born in Musquodoboit Harbour, Halifax County, d/o Simeon and Christie (Dares) Gates, Preston, Halifax County, she was nursing in Halifax and had more than two years' CAMC experience when she joined the CAMCNS in April 1918. She served in No. 10 CGH, No. 2 CCCS and No. 16 CGH until being SOS in March 1919. She married John Swim, a Lockeport seafood merchant in November 1919. They later lived in Liverpool, Queens County, but are buried in Yarmouth.

104. Genders, Sarah Elizabeth (1890–1990). Born in London, England, d/o John and Elizabeth (Wileman) Genders, Milford Station, Hants County, she was living in Halifax and had CAMC experience when she joined the CAMCNS in December 1916. She served in No. 1 CGH and No. 8 CGH and in 1923 was awarded the French Médaille d'honneur des Epidemies en Vermeil, which honoured people who had distinguished themselves by their dedication during epidemic diseases.[216] In August 1919 she returned to Halifax and served in CHH and CMH until being demobilized in August 1920. She then moved to Newport, Rhode Island, where she worked as a private nurse and applied for social security in 1951 but is buried in the Milford Cemetery, Milford Station. Her brother, John Genders, enlisted in the 246th Battalion in May 1917 but served overseas in the 185th Battalion and the 2nd Battalion Canadian Machine Gun Corps.

105. Gilbert, Phyllis Nora (1892–1972). Born in Halifax, Halifax County, d/o Walter and Sarah Jane "Daisy" (Lillywhite) Gilbert, who had emigrated to Halifax in 1888, then moved to Montreal, later to Medicine Hat, Alberta, and finally to Calgary in 1903,[217] she trained at Holy Cross General Hospital and had three years' CAMC experience when she joined the CAMCNS in Edmonton in March 1917. She served in the Kitchener Military Hospital and No. 10 CGH but fell ill with influenza and neurasthenia and was invalided home in November 1917. She then served in the Calgary General Hospital and Strathcona Military Hospital in Edmonton until being SOS as "medically unfit" in December 1918. According to her obituary, however, she resumed nursing at Holy Cross until her retirement.[218]

106. Gilchrist, Marion Leigh (1891–1963). Born in Necum Teuch, Halifax County, d/o William and Mary (Parker) Gilchrist, she and her family moved to Saskatchewan in 1906, then to Vidora, a village near Moose Jaw. She had returned to Halifax, however, and was nursing with two months' CAMC experience when she joined the CAMCNS in July 1918. She was sent overseas but fell ill and was transferred to Halifax, where she served in CHH

and subsidiaries from January to June 1919, when she was SOS. She then moved to Maple Creek, Saskatchewan, to live with her brother Reuben and his wife in 1921, but was living in Medicine Hat, Alberta, in 1931 and died there. Another brother, John Gilchrist, was conscripted into the Saskatchewan Regiment at Regina in August 1918 but died of pneumonia in December 1918.

107. Gillis, Christine Anna (1885–1960). Born in Sydney Forks, Cape Breton, d/o Joseph and Katie (MacKinnon) (deceased) Gillis, she was nursing in Halifax and had four months' CAMC experience when she shaved four years from her date of birth and joined the CAMCNS in August 1918. She served with the MD 6 Training Depot, the CHH and subsidiary facilities until being SOS in March 1919. Two years later she moved to Quincy, Massachusetts, and married John Angus Gillis, a carpenter from Inverness, Cape Breton, in 1922. They later lived in Somerville, Massachusetts.

108. Godard, Alice Maude (1884–1960). Born in Passaic, New Jersey, d/o Cyprian and Sarah (Gelling) Godard, she had studied nursing in the United States and worked there until the family moved to Bridgewater, Nova Scotia. She nursed there and had CAMC experience when she joined the CAMCNS in May 1917. She served with the DCRC, No. 15 CGH, No. 8 CGH, No. 11 CGH, No. 9 CGH and No. 16 CGH. She returned home in August 1919 and was demobilized in September 1919, then worked briefly in Halifax. She then returned to Hackensack, New Jersey, as a public health nurse, but in 1940 retired to Halifax. Her brother, Arthur Godard, enlisted in the 55th Battalion but served overseas in the 25th Battalion and died of wounds received at Vimy Ridge.

109. Graham, Catherine Mary (1871–1959). Born in Halifax, Halifax County, d/o John and Bridget (Fahie) Graham, she was an 1895 graduate of the VGH School of Nursing and completed postgraduate courses in public health at Dalhousie University and pediatrics at the Blossom Street Infants' Hospital in Boston. She had four years' CAMC experience in the CMH and named her sister, Ella Maud Graham, as NOK when she joined CAMCNS in June 1918, shaving seven years off her date of birth. She went overseas and was appointed nursing supervisor at No. 16 CGH in Orpington, Kent, England. She returned to Halifax in August 1918, served in the CMH, and was acting matron of the Pine Hill Convalescent Hospital. After demobilization she continued nursing at CHH and also served as matron of Rainbow Haven Camp at Cole Harbour, Halifax County, a summer camp for underprivileged children. She served as president of the Halifax branch and provincial president three times in 1917–1918, 1921 and 1928–1930 and was also the first president of the GNANS, when registered nurses obtained their RN

designation in 1922. In 2009 the College of Registered Nurses of Nova Scotia awarded her posthumously with the Centennial Award of Distinction for her contribution to the nursing profession.

110. Graham, Harriet (1883–1932). Born in New Glasgow, Pictou County, d/o Harvey and Hannah (Fraser) Graham (both deceased), and stepdaughter of Emma (MacKay) Graham and a cousin of Pearl Fraser (*See* #98). Her father was a prominent industrialist with the Nova Scotia Steel and Coal Company in New Glasgow. She was a 1914 graduate of the St. Luke's Hospital School of Nursing in New York and immediately joined the CAMCNS in Quebec in September 1914. She served in No. 2 CSH, No. 11 CGH, No. 2 CCCS and No. 10 CSH and was awarded the Royal Red Cross 2nd Class in June 1917. She was promoted to matron of the Canadian Officers' Red Cross Hospital in London in April 1918 and may have served two years as matron of a military hospital at Burlington, Ontario,[219] then the Davisville Orthopaedic Military Hospital in Toronto in May 1919. She was nursing in New Glasgow when she married James Macdonald, a businessman in La Prairie, Saskatchewan, in 1924. They later lived in Saskatoon, although she died in Victoria, BC.

111. Grant, Grace Mabel (1885–1919). Born in Halifax, Halifax County, d/o John (deceased) and Isabel Ellen (Umlah) Grant, she was a 1903 graduate of the VGH School of Nursing and worked in a small hospital at Somerville, Maine, until returning to Halifax in November 1916. She joined the CAMCNS in March 1918 and served with the MD 6 Training Depot and CHH until falling ill with influenza in October 1918. She was transferred to a staff position with the acting director of Medical Services until April 1919 when she was posted to CHH but then was admitted to CMH and died in September 1919. Her brother, Horace Belford Grant, served as a lieutenant in the 27th Battalion and was killed in action in August 1917.

112. Grant, Janie (1871–1956). Born in Sunny Brae, Pictou County, d/o John and Margaret (MacIntosh) Grant, she studied nursing in Providence, Rhode Island, and worked as a private nurse there until joining the United States Navy in May 1918. She served at the US Navy No. 1 Base Hospital in Brest, France, in November 1917, the first US Naval Base hospital fully equipped for the American Expeditionary Forces. She was SOS when it was disestablished in 1919 and resumed nursing in Providence until about 1931 when she returned home to Sunny Brae.

113. Grattan, Rosanna "Myrtle" (1887–1966). Born in Moncton, New Brunswick, d/o John and Margaret (Hannigan) Grattan, who were originally from Pictou, Pictou County, she was a graduate of the Roosevelt Hospital School of Nursing in New York and was working there when she joined the CAMCNS. She served in No. 1 CGH in Quebec City in September 1914 and

in No. 2 CSH at Le Touquet until resigning in February 1916 and being sent home because she had become pregnant. Meanwhile, Dr. Charles Andrew Young, an Ottawa physician also serving in No. 2 CSH had suffered a series of health issues, which enabled him to return home "on duty" in January 1916. A month later they married in Pictou, after which he returned overseas, and Myrtle (and the baby) lived with his mother in Ottawa. He rose to the rank of temporary lieutenant colonel in March 1918 and was mentioned in dispatches but fell ill again with appendicitis and influenza in the spring of 1919 and was SOS. By 1921 he had recovered and another baby was born in 1920. Charles returned to Ottawa where he continued practising medicine and died in 1959.

114. Graves, Laura May (1890–1968). Born in Halifax, Halifax County, d/o Noah and Sarah (Cunningham) Graves, she was a 1915 graduate of the VGH School of Nursing and had two years seven months' CAMC experience with the MD 6 Training Depot when she joined the CAMCNS in August 1918. She served in CHH and at Camp Aldershot from October 1918 to August 1919, when she was demobilized. She continued nursing in Halifax until retiring in 1937. Her father died on December 9, 1917, of injuries received in the Halifax Explosion.

115. Gray, Dorothy "Dora" Louise (1883–1942). Born in Stellarton, Pictou County, d/o Alexander and Agnes (Whyte) Gray, New Glasgow, and sister of Marguerite Olive Gray (*See* #116), she was a graduate of Beth Israel Hospital in Roxbury, Massachusetts. She joined the CAMCNS in Halifax in September 1915 and served with No. 5 CGH and No. 1 CGH until being transferred to England because of health issues and being invalided home in July 1919. She was demobilized in October 1919 and later lived in Los Angeles and died there in 1942.

116. Gray, Marguerite Olive (1885–1949). Born in New Glasgow, Pictou County, d/o Alexander and Agnes (Whyte) Gray and sister of Dorothy Gray (*See* #115), she had nine months' experience with the Harvard Surgical Unit in RAMC No. 22 Hospital at Camiers until joining the CEF in London in April 1916. She served in the Granville Canadian Special Hospital at Ramsgate, No. 1 CSH at Salonika, where she was awarded the Royal Red Cross 2nd Class, and No. 10 CGH in Kitchener, England. She returned home in December 1918 because of health issues and was SOS in April 1919, so she returned to New Glasgow and became a public health nurse.

117. Guild, Effie Jean (1893–1956). Born in Head of Chezzetcook, Halifax County, d/o George and Lydia (Semple) Guild, she was a 1915 graduate of the VGH School of Nursing, was nursing in Halifax and had CAMC experience when she shaved three years off and joined the CAMCNS in December 1917. She

served in No. 14 CGH, No. 13 CGH and No. 10 CSH, returning to Halifax in May 1919, where she nursed briefly at CHH and subsidiaries until being SOS in August 1919. She resumed nursing at the VGH and, in about 1930, married Dr. Robert Harvey Stoddard, a Halifax physician, who was from Clam Harbour, a village close to Head of Chezzetcook, and continued nursing until 1953.

118. Gunn, Elva Maud (1885–1938). Born in Gore, Hants County, d/o Adam (deceased) and Susan (McLellan) Gunn, and a cousin of Mary Catherine Gunn, she was a 1911 graduate of the Western Hospital School of Nursing in London, Ontario.[220] She had two and a half years' experience in private nursing in 1916 when she briefly served at the Hugh Waddell Memorial Hospital in Canora, Saskatchewan. In October 1916 she went to England and joined the QAIMNS, serving at Birmingham's War Hospital No. 1. A year later she transferred into the CAMCNS in London and served in No. 11 CGH until falling ill with influenza, and No. 9 CGH at Kinmel Park, until being SOS and returning home in July 1919. She then took six months of hospital retraining and a nursing course at Winnipeg's Margaret Scott Nursing Mission and was one of the Manitoba Division of the Canadian Red Cross Society's first two nurses to serve in remote nursing stations. Her brother, William Gunn, enlisted in the 196th (Winnipeg) Battalion at the age of sixteen and but was transferred into the 128th (Moose Jaw) Battalion but then fell ill with tuberculosis and was SOS in May 1917.

119. Gunn, Mary Catherine Nichols (1886–1979). Born in East River, Pictou County, d/o William and Margaret (MacInnis) Gunn, and a cousin of Elva Maud Gunn, she studied nursing in Seattle, Washington, and gave an address in Calgary when shaved three years from her date of birth and joined the CAMCNS in January 1917. Although she had been serving at a temporary military hospital in Lethbridge, Alberta, she served with the DCRC, No. 1 CGH, No. 8 CGH, No. 5 CCCS, No. 2 CSH, No. 5 CCCS, No. 11 CGH, No. 12 CGH and No. 16 CGH until being sent home because of health issues and was SOS in August 1919. She returned to Calgary and became a public health nurse. When she retired in 1952, the Calgary Board of Education named a school in her honour.

120. Haliburton, Marion Frances (1888–1969). Born in Halifax, Halifax County, d/o Alfred and Katherine (Donovan) Haliburton and a descendant of T. C. Haliburton, the famous Nova Scotian author, she was a 1915 graduate of the Université Laval School of Nursing and joined No. 6 (Laval) CGH in Quebec City in December 1915. She served in the Moore Barracks Hospital at Shorncliffe, later designated No. 11 CGH; the Hôpital Temporaire d'Arc-en-Barrois, a civilian British hospital established by the British

Red Cross under the military command of the French army's Service de Santé des Armées; No. 2 CGH; and No. 12 CGH but struggled with health issues and returned to Halifax in September 1918. She then served at CHH and subsidiaries until being SOS in May 1919, after which she continued nursing in Halifax until her retirement in 1953. She served as president of the Registered Nurses' Association of Nova Scotia (RNANS) in 1937–38. Two of her brothers, Alfred and Arthur, were officers in the Canadian Garrison Artillery during the war, and a nephew, William Alfred Haliburton, served in RAF Coastal Command during the Second World War and was killed in May 1942.

121. Hallisey, Kathleen Martina (1890–1989). Born in Truro, Colchester County, d/o John and Mary Catherine (Carroll) Hallisey, she was nursing in Halifax when she joined the CAMCNS in April 1918. She was posted to No. 15. CGH but soon fell ill and was in hospital for two months, then returned to Halifax and was SOS in June 1919. In November 1919 she married Leveson Gower Fraser, a son of Rose and Mary Lewis (Masters) Fraser, who was conscripted in October 1917 and served in No. 10 Halifax Siege Battery during the war. They lived in Truro and later Halifax. Her brother, John Hallisey, served as a lieutenant in Nova Scotia's 25th Battalion and was killed at Vimy Ridge.

122. Hamm, Lila Agnes. *See* Donovan, Lila Agnes.

123. Hare, Olla Dell. *See* Lester, Olla Dell.

124. Harlow, Harriett "Hattie" Amelia (1893–1929). Born in North Brookfield, Queens County, d/o Maurice Almon and Dora (Waterman) Harlow, Bridgewater, Lunenburg County, she attended the Acadia University Seminary (collegiate course), graduating in 1912. She appears to have studied nursing in New England or New York because she joined the Harvard Surgical Unit and likely served at RAMC No. 22 General Hospital in Étaples. She may have served also with one of the Canadian military hospitals on Lemnos, which likely explains how she met Lieutenant Reginald Dale Boyes, an England-born lawyer from Auckland, New Zealand, when most of the New Zealand troops at Gallipoli evacuated to Lemnos. They moved to Auckland and married in 1920. Her brother, Albert Harlow, served in the 25th Battalion and was killed at Ypres on November 8, 1917.

125. Harrison, Eunice Knapp (1883–1975). Born in Southampton, Cumberland County, d/o Moses (deceased) and Matilda (Davidson) Harrison, she was nursing in nearby Nappan but appears to have gone to England in 1915 and joined the QAIMNS. She served at the Lord Derby War Hospital in Warrington, Lancashire County, a former psychiatric hospital. She transferred into the CAMCNS in London in December 1917 and served in No. 15 CGH, on the *Araguaya* hospital ship, and the Canadian Eye and Ear Hospital at

Shorncliffe, then was attached to a British unit in France, No. 3 CSH, No. 8 CSH and the CCCS at Bexhill. In June 1919 she returned to Halifax and served at CHH and subsidiaries until being demobilized in January 1920. In about 1960 she married Frederick Le Mottee, a son of Colonel John Le Mottee, brother of Rear Admiral Douglas Balfour Le Mottee, nephew of Lieutenant Colonel Henry Le Mottee, and brother of Major Edward D'Albret Le Mottee, Guernsey Islands. He had visited Canada on a number of occasions but immigrated in 1925 and lived in Toronto, then Victoria, BC, where his first wife died in 1957. He died in 1971.

126. Harrison, Jean Augusta (1885[221]–1966). Born in Amherst, Cumberland County, d/o Albert and Edith (Fuller) Harrison, Maccan, Cumberland County, she had served as head nurse in a hospital in Iowa City, Iowa, in 1915 but was nursing in Winnipeg when she joined the CEF in March 1917. She served with the CAMC Training Depot at Shorncliffe, the DCRC, No. 2 CGH, No. 6 CGH and No. 11 CGH, returning home in June 1919. She was living with her brother, Elton Harrison, at River Hebert, Cumberland County, in 1921 but then moved to Winnipeg and perhaps Lloydminster, Alberta, where in 1924 she married Robert Tomlinson, an American from Minnesota. They lived in nearby Innisfree in 1946. She died less than a month after participating in Innisfree's 1966 Remembrance Day commemoration.[222] Her brother, Fletcher Harrison, who lived in Saskatoon, Saskatchewan, served briefly in the 95th Battalion and the Canadian Forestry Corps in England.

127. Hartling, Mabel Etta (1887–1964). Born in Port Dufferin, Halifax County, d/o William Reuben and Agnes (Ives) Hartling, she was a 1912 graduate of the VGH School of Nursing and nursed with the VON for a year, then joined the CAMC and served at the CMH. In June 1918 she joined the CAMCNS and served in No. 9 CGH at Shorncliffe and No. 4 CGH until falling ill and was invalided to Halifax in May 1919. She served briefly in CMH again until being SOS as "medically unfit" in August 1919, although she did private duty nursing until retiring in 1953. Two of her brothers, Aubrey and Duncan, served in the war: Aubrey in the 25th Battalion, and Duncan, who had moved to Edmonton, in the 50th Battalion, and both were wounded in 1917.

128. Haverstock, Laura Grace (1880–1964). Born in Halifax, Halifax County, d/o James and Caroline (Melvin) Haverstock, she had seven months' CAMC experience when she joined the CAMCNS in July 1918. She served in the MD 6 Training Depot and CHH and subsidiary hospitals until being SOS in August 1919. She continued nursing in Halifax until retiring in 1929. Her brother, Roy Haverstock, who was already a member of the 8th Siege Battery at Halifax, was conscripted in April 1918 and served in the 6th Siege Battery Artillery at Halifax.

129. Hayden, Mary Josephine (1877–1952). Born in Halifax, Halifax County, d/o John and Johannah (Walsh) Hayden, she may have studied nursing at Roxbury, Massachusetts, because she named her sister-in-law, the wife of her brother, James Hayden, who lived there, as NOK. She was nursing in Halifax and had twenty-nine months' CAMC experience when she joined the CAMCNS in July 1918. She served in the MD 6 Training Depot, CHH and subsidiaries until being SOS in August 1919. She was nursing in Halifax in 1925 but retired in 1939.[223]

130. Hillcoat, Anna "Annie" Rebecca (1880–1942). Born in Darnley, PEI, d/o Dr. Hedley Vicars Hillcoat, a veterinarian surgeon, and Elizabeth (McArthur) Hillcoat, Amherst, Cumberland County, she studied nursing at the Connecticut Training School for Nurses in Hartford, Connecticut, and completed a graduate course at Johns Hopkins Hospital in Baltimore. She nursed in the Hartford Hospital and claimed to have CAMC experience when she shaved seven years from her date of birth to join the CAMCNS in Montreal in July 1918. She served in No. 16 CGH until falling ill and being invalided in May 1918 to Halifax, where she served with the MD 6 Casualty Hospital and Training Depot. In October 1918 she transferred to the Charlottetown Military Hospital as matron but returned to Halifax in May 1919 to serve at CHH and subsidiaries until being SOS in January 1920. She was superintendent of nurses at the Highland View Hospital in Amherst when she died. Her brother, Hedley Vicars Hillcoat, was conscripted in October 1917 and served in the 17th Reserve Battalion at Bramshott Camp but returned home in July 1919 after being diagnosed with rheumatic myalgia.

131. Hogan, Elizabeth Cecilia. *See* Doyle, Elizabeth Cecilia.

132. Howard, Alice Maud (1891–1989). Born in Montreal, Quebec, d/o Martin and Lydia (Young) Howard, Guysborough, Guysborough County, she was living in Edmonton when she joined the CAMCNS in Montreal in June 1915. She served overseas in No. 1 CGH, No. 2 CGH and the Westcliffe Canadian Eye and Ear Hospital, then was transferred to Halifax in January 1919 and served briefly at CHH until being discharged in March 1919. She returned to Edmonton and nursed at the University Hospital. In 1927 she married Francis Connors, a civil engineer from Chatham, New Brunswick. He had enlisted in the 12th Canadian Mounted Rifles in January 1915 but served overseas with the Canadian Railway Construction Corps with the rank of captain until developing health issues and was SOS in July 1918 as "medically unfit." After his death in 1966, she moved to Kamloops, British Columbia. Her brother, Douglas Howard, joined the 85th Battalion in October 1915 and was gassed during the Battle of Valenciennes in November 1918.

133. Howe, Fanny "Myrtle" (1883–1966). Born in Nictaux, Annapolis County, d/o Sydenham and Fanny (Westphal) Howe, and granddaughter of Joseph Howe, she was a 1916 graduate of the VGH School of Nursing and served overseas in the QAIMNS, then returned to Nictaux but died in Halifax. Her brother, John Ross Howe, was manager and agent of Sun Life of Canada Insurance Company in Kingston, Jamaica, until enlisting as a staff sergeant in the British West Indies Regiment in 1915, then company quartermaster sergeant in its second battalion, but died in Kingston in June 1918.[224]

134. Hubley, Janet "Jennie" Mabel (1883–1970). Born in Halifax, Halifax County, d/o Silas (deceased) and Emma (Langille) Hubley,[225] she was a 1908 graduate of the VGH School of Nursing, nursed in Bar Harbor, Maine, for a year and then was night supervisor in a hospital in Atlantic City but returned home because of illness in her family. She then nursed in Halifax and had fifteen months' CAMC experience when she shaved four years from her date of birth to join the CAMCNS in May 1917. She served in No. 10 CSH, No. 14 CGH and No. 11 CGH, then was sent home in December 1918 because of health issues. She served with the MD 6 Training Unit and CHH and subsidiaries until being SOS in August 1919. She studied public health nursing at Dalhousie University and nursed in the Dalhousie Public Health Clinic for twenty-five years, retiring in 1966.

135. Hubley, Laura May (1875–1964). Born in St. Margaret's Bay, Halifax County, d/o Robert and Jane (deceased) Hubley and stepdaughter of Carrie (Innis) Hubley, she was an 1898 graduate of the VGH School of Nursing and went into private practice in Halifax until 1912, when she joined the CAMC and nursed in the CMH and Rockhead Military Hospital. In November 1915 she shaved three years from her date of birth and listed her aunt, Jessie Hubley, as her NOK when she joined the CAMCNS. She served as matron of No. 7 CSH and also in No. 3 CGH, No. 8 CSH, the Westcliffe Canadian Eye and Ear Hospital, and the Buxton's Canadian Red Cross Special Hospital. She was awarded the Royal Red Cross 1st Class and represented Matron-in-Chief Margaret Macdonald at the national thanksgiving of peace ceremony in St. Paul's Cathedral, London, in July 1919 with the King and Queen and Princess Louise, the Duchess of Argyll, present.[226] She then returned home and served as matron of the CMH at CHH in Halifax. She was the president

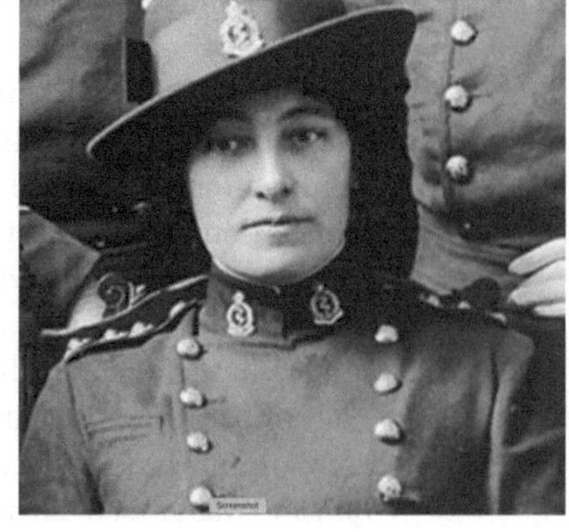

Laura May Hubley. [WIKITREE.COM]

of the GNANS from 1923 to 1926, when it changed its name to the Registered Nurses' Association of Nova Scotia (RNANS) and introduced the first RN provincial examinations. She was also a member of the committee that planned the national memorial in the parliament building to Canadian nurses who died in the war. She later was transferred to a military hospital in London, Ontario, retiring in Halifax in 1938. In 2009 the College of Registered Nurses of Nova Scotia posthumously awarded her the Centennial Award of Distinction for her contribution to nursing.

136. Hunt, Minnie Hannah (1877–1969). Born in Mabou, Inverness County, d/o Joseph and Rachel (Frizzle) Hunt (deceased) and sister of Myrtle Margaret Hunt (*See* #137), she lived in Los Angeles from 1914 to 1917 and served in the American Red Cross Children's Hospital at Evian, France,[227] until shaving three years off her date of birth and joining the CAMCNS in London in June 1918. She served in No. 13 CGH and No. 16 CGH, returned home in July 1919 and was SOS in August 1919. She may have moved to Australia but was nursing in Vancouver, BC, in 1940 and died there.

137. Hunt, Myrtle Margaret (1884–1918). Born in Mabou, Inverness County, d/o Joseph and Rachel (Frizzle) Hunt (deceased) and sister of Minnie Hannah Hunt (*See* #136), she was a graduate of the VGH School of Nursing and nursed at the Halifax Infirmary, a hospital operated by the Sisters of Charity of Saint Vincent de Paul, until dying of pneumonia complicated by nephritis in January 1918.[228] Although she didn't join the CAMC or the CAMCNS, her death certificate in the Nova Scotia Archives describes her as "Nurse Military Hospital,"[229] her tombstone is an official Commonwealth War Graves marker, and the Canadian Virtual War Memorial includes her on its website.[230]

138. Irwin, Eliza "Blanche" (1882–1956). Born in Wine Harbour, Guysborough County, d/o George (deceased) and Annie (McCutcheon) Irwin, she had fifteen months' CAMC experience when she shaved a year off her date of birth and joined the CAMCNS in September 1917. She nursed at the Moxham Castle and Ross Convalescent Hospitals in Sydney, Cape Breton, until being demobilized in January 1919. In 1921 she was living with her mother and working as a private nurse. She subsequently married Hayden Rood, a millwright from Port Hilford, Guysborough County, who had been living in Kirkland Lake, Ontario, when he was conscripted in Toronto in April 1918. He arrived in England in October 1918 and briefly served as a sapper with the Canadian Engineers until being posted to the notorious Kinmel Park, holding camp in Wales in January 1919. After he was discharged to Toronto in July 1919, they married and moved to northern Ontario, where he was superintendent of the Lake Shore Mine at Kirkland Lake.

139. Jaggard, Jessie Brown (1873–1915). Born in Wolfville, Kings County, d/o John and Elizabeth (Whidden) Brown and a cousin of Robert Borden, she attended the Acadia University Seminary (collegiate course), then trained at the McLean Hospital and Massachusetts General Hospital in Boston. She became assistant superintendent of the Norristown State Hospital in Philadelphia and, later, University of Pennsylvania Hospital in Philadelphia. There she met and married Herbert Jaggard, a graduate of Yale University who was general agent of the Pennsylvania Railroad's lines west of Pittsburgh. Although over age, she joined the CAMCNS in London, England, was appointed matron of No. 3 CSH's nurses in April 1915 and went with the unit to Lemnos in August 1915. She and another nurse, Mary Munro, from Niagara-on-the-Lake in Ontario, died there of dysentery in September 1915 and were buried in the Portianou Military Cemetery. Her husband and mother each received the Memorial Cross for her sacrifice in 1921.[231] She is commemorated on a memorial tablet in the Massachusetts General Hospital School of Nursing.[232] When Vera Brittain, the British poet who was serving as a VAD on HMHS *Britannic*, visited Lemnos in 1916 and saw their graves, she wrote a poem, "The Sisters' Graves at Lemnos," (*See* page 41) which was published in the *Oxford Magazine* (May 11, 1917) and in *Poems of the War and After* (1934).

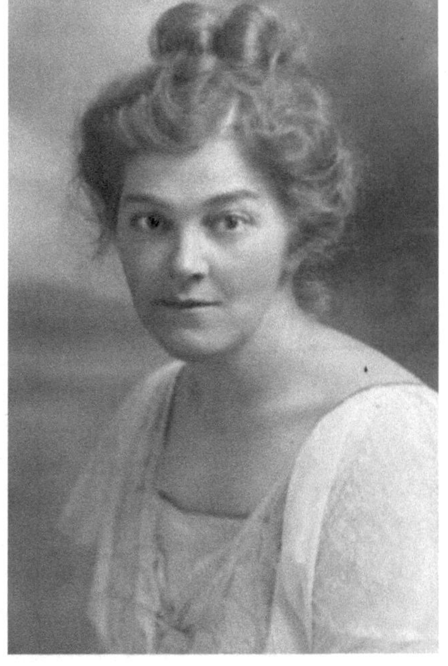
Jessie Jaggard. [COMMONWEALTH WAR GRAVES COMMISSION]

140. Jarvis, Jessie Agnes McCully (1888–1918). Born in Moncton, New Brunswick, d/o George (deceased) and Frances (McCully) Jarvis, she and her mother and sister moved to Truro, Colchester County. She trained at the Worcester City Hospital in Massachusetts and nursed there before returning home in 1914 and nursing there. In October 1917 she joined the CAMCNS in Halifax and served in the CMH until dying of pneumonia on May 23, 1918. Her brother, Ralph Jarvis, was conscripted in October 1917 and served with No. 9 Siege Battery in Saint John.

141. Jenner, Lenna Mae (1889–1918). Born in North Brookfield, Queens County, d/o Rev. John Hugh and Mary Fisher (MacIntyre) Jenner, Saint John, New

Brunswick, she was a 1913 graduate of the Winnipeg General Hospital School of Nursing and was nursing in the Saint John General Public Hospital in New Brunswick. She had fourteen months' CMH experience when she went to Halifax and joined the CAMCNS in June 1918.[233] She was sent to England in July and served briefly in the Westcliffe Canadian Eye and Ear Hospital until falling ill with septicaemia in October 1918. She died in the Barnet Military Hospital in Barnet, Hertfordshire, in December 1918. In 1921 a memorial room in the Saint John General Public Hospital's Nurses' Home was named in her honour. Her father was a Baptist minister who had attended Acadia University and the Newton Seminary in Springfield, Massachusetts, before returning to Nova Scotia. Her brother, Hugh Jenner, served in Nova Scotia's 25th Battalion and the No. 2 Motor Machine Gun Brigade.

142. Johnston, Alice Mary (1883–1967). Born in Bridgeport (Dominion), Cape Breton, d/o Prescott and Alice (Hare) Johnston, Dartmouth, Halifax County, she was a great-granddaughter of James William Johnston, a lawyer and politician who served as premier of Nova Scotia in 1857–60 and 1863–4 and was briefly lieutenant governor. Her uncle, Arthur Clement Johnston, mayor of Dartmouth in 1891–97, sold the family's large Mount Amelia estate, retaining only the home on Pleasant Street in Dartmouth, to which Johnston's family moved after managing a family-owned coal mine in Bridgeport. The house is now a designated heritage property.[234] Alice was a graduate of the St. Joseph's Hospital School of Nursing and went to England, serving briefly with RAMC No. 2 Stationary Hospital, then transferred into the CEF and served in No. 7 CSH and No. 8 CGH. She returned home in May 1919 and served in CHH and CMH. Upon being SOS in June 1920, she moved to Bermuda, where her sister, Edith Johnston, lived, to serve as matron at the King Edward VII Memorial Hospital, but returned home in 1924 and was serving in the Rockhead Isolation Hospital, Halifax, in 1924–25. Her older brother, James William Johnston, enlisted in the 9th Battalion at Valcartier in September 1914 but served overseas in the 2nd Battalion, was wounded in June 1915 and killed in action in February 1916. Her younger brother, Cyril Preston Johnston, then enlisted in the 6th Overseas Universities Company but served with the Princess Patricia's Canadian Light Infantry until falling ill in January 1918. He was treated in England and attached to No. 6 Canadian Reserve Battalion until being SOS in February 1919.

143. Jones, Helen Lorna (1895–1974). Born in Ithaca, New York, d/o Howard Parker and Elizabeth Isabel (Ridd) Jones, Dartmouth, Halifax County, she had VAD experience in England at the Gifford House Hospital and Leicester Base Hospital but apparently was a trained nurse because she trans-

ferred into the CAMCNS in London in June 1917. She served in the Monks Horton Convalescent Hospital at Westenhanger near Folkestone in Kent and the Kitchener Military Convalescent Hospital until developing health issues and returned home in January 1919. In 1920 she married Richard Roome, a Dartmouth jeweller, who had served in the Royal Canadian Artillery but transferred into the Royal Field Artillery in September 1915, serving in France, India and Mesopotamia. After the war he co-founded Harris and Roome Ltd, a wholesale distribution company specializing in electrical items, hardware, and batteries, and was active in the militia. In the Second World War he returned to active duty, commanding the 5th Field Regiment of the Royal Canadian Artillery until being promoted to brigadier general commanding 7th Division Artillery in Eastern Canada, then was posted to Defence Headquarters in Ottawa, was promoted to deputy adjutant general, and in 1945 was awarded the Commander of the British Empire (CBE) medal for his service. His papers are housed in the Dalhousie University Archives and the Nova Scotia Archives.[235]

144. Keith, Gertrude Jane (1883–1971). Born in Halifax, Halifax County, d/o Samuel and Ella (Knight) Keith, she was a 1912 graduate of the VGH School of Nursing and was a head nurse at the VGH until 1913. She had fourteen months' CAMC experience in the CMH when she joined the CAMCNS in July 1918. She served in CMH and CHH but experienced health issues including tonsilitis, influenza and appendicitis and was discharged as "medically unfit" in January 1919. She was the first secretary of the VGH School of Nursing Alumnae Association when it was founded in 1920, married Frederick Smith McLellan, a contractor, in June 1920, and continued nursing until 1965.

145. Kendall, Helen Mary (1892–1957). Born in Sydney, Cape Breton, d/o Dr. Henry and Ida (Burchell) (deceased) Kendall, Halifax, stepdaughter of Margaret McLennan and half-sister of Katharine McLennan, she was a 1916 graduate of the RVH School of Nursing in Montreal, where she studied surgical nursing and was one of the first nurses trained as an anaesthetist. She had CAMC experience with the CMH in Halifax when she joined the CAMCNS in January 1917. She went overseas in March 1917 on the *Essequibo*, a hospital ship that was stopped by U-54, a German submarine, but was allowed to continue on its way. She served in No. 16 CGH, the Canadian Forestry Corps Hospital at Lajoux, and No. 2 CGH, where she took an anaesthesia course. She was serving in No. 7 CGH when it was bombed by German aircraft in May 1918 and was awarded the Royal Red Cross 2nd Class for her exceptional service. She also served in No. 3 CSH and No. 5 CGH. She returned home in October 1919, resumed nursing at the RVH,

and was one of the first nurse anaesthetists there.[236] She was then one of the eight members of a Canadian Nursing Mission led by Dorothy P. Cotton that went to Bucharest, Romania, in 1920 to establish a school of nursing at Cotzea Hospital.[237] She served again in No. 1 Canadian Neurological Hospital and as sister in charge in No. 4 CCCS in England in the early part of the Second World War, returning to the RVH in Montreal in 1942. Her father, who was a physician, joined No. 9 CSH and commanded it from 1916 to 1918 and later served as lieutenant governor of Nova Scotia. His brother, Arthur Kendall, was also a physician but also served in the Nova Scotia House of Assembly from 1897 to 1900 and 1904 to 1911, and in the House of Commons from 1901 to 1904.

146. Kennedy, Margaret Evelyn (1888–1954). Born in Musquodoboit Harbour, Halifax County, d/o Edward (deceased) and Marguerite (Smith) Kennedy and stepdaughter of Parker Archibald, Halifax, she was nursing in the Nova Scotia Hospital in 1911[238] and had thirty months' CAMC experience, including the Halifax Explosion, when she shaved two years off her date of birth and joined the CAMCNS in July 1918. She served in Halifax at CMH and CHH until injuring her back and being SOS in February 1919. She was practising private nursing and living with her parents in 1921.

147. Killam, Annie Maud (1890–1991). Born in Scott Settlement, New Brunswick, d/o Martin and Mary (Fairweather) Killam, Tusket, Yarmouth County, she studied nursing in Worcester, Massachusetts, and served with the American Red Cross in the war. In 1926 she married Harrison Hill, a civil engineer from Litchfield, Connecticut, and they lived in Norwalk, Wethersfield, and Hartford, Connecticut. She is commemorated on Tusket's war memorial. Her brother, Scott Killam, enlisted in the 219th Battalion but served in the 85th Battalion and was wounded in September 1918.

148. King, Hazel May (1885–1967). Born in Annapolis Royal, Annapolis County, d/o Arthur and Mary (Goldsmith) King, she had a year's experience in France with the Harvard Surgical Unit at No. 4 RAMC Hospital when she transferred to the CAMCNS in London in June 1917. She served in the Kitchener Military Hospital (redesignated No. 10 CGH in September 1917) and the Canadian Red Cross Officers Hospital in London until falling ill and being SOS in July 1919. In 1920 she married John Bell, a veteran who was born in New Brunswick but was living in Toronto when he joined the 124th Battalion with the rank of captain and served overseas with the 12th Battalion Canadian Engineers. They lived in Toronto.

149. Landells, Margaret Jane "Jean" (1879–1957). Born in Cooks Brook, Halifax County, d/o George and Ann (Kerr) Landells, she had CAMC experience and served for a year with the British Red Cross before transferring to the CAMCNS in London in June 1916. She served in No. 1 CSH and No. 4

CGH at Salonika, then No. 12 CGH at Bramshott and contracted measles and nephritis. She returned to Halifax in July 1919 and served at CHH and CMH from September 1919 to February 1920. After the war she earned a postgraduate certificate in surgery, pediatrics and obstetrics at Bellevue Hospital, New York. She subsequently moved to Lloydminster, Alberta, and married William Roebuck, a local farmer, but after his death returned to Nova Scotia and nursed in Truro until retiring to Musquodoboit Harbour.

150. LaPierre, Mary Anna (1889–1929). Born in Halifax, Halifax County, d/o Rufus and Catherine Lapierre, Dartmouth, she had two months' CAMC experience when she joined the CAMCNS in July 1918. She served in Halifax in the CMH and CHH until being demobilized in July 1919. In 1920 she married Dr. Ernest Fraser Moore, a Halifax physician who had eight years' CAMC experience with No. 1 Field Ambulance when he joined the CAMC in November 1918 and served at CHH until January 1920. They later lived at Canso, Guysborough County.

151. Larkin, Nora Evelyn (1883–1955). Born in Tipperary, Ireland, d/o Matthew (deceased) and Bridget Mae (Doherty) Larkin, and immigrated to Nova Scotia in 1895, she was a 1911 graduate of the VGH School of Nursing and had seventeen months' CAMC experience in the CMH when shaved two years from her date of birth and joined the CAMCNS in July 1918. She served at CMH and CHH until being SOS in September 1919. She continued nursing until about 1950.

152. Layton, Adriana Robertson (1884–1966). Born in Elmsdale, Hants County, d/o Rev. Jacob and Margaret (Smith) Layton, Oakfield, Halifax County, she had nine months' CAMC experience at Camp Aldershot and was recommended by Lieutenant Colonel Joseph Hayes for promotion to matron of the camp hospital but was not approved by military authorities.[239] In December 1916 she joined the CAMCNS, naming her sister, Anne Layton, as NOK. She served in No. 9 CGH, No. 8 CSH and No. 1 CGH until developing health issues that resulted in her being returned to Halifax for medical treatment. She served in the MD 6 Casualty Hospital and Training Depot until being SOS in December 1918. In 1920 she married James Murphy, a blacksmith, and they lived in Brookfield, Colchester County. After his death in 1942, she moved to New Westminster, British Columbia, and married George Simmons in 1948.[240]

153. LeJeune, Marie[241] Catherine (1893–?). Born in West Arichat, Richmond County, d/o William and Marie LeJeune, she was living in Halifax and had ten months' CAMC experience at the Moxham Castle Convalescent Hospital in Sydney when she shaved two years off her date of birth to join the CAMCNS in October 1918, naming her sister, Delvina LeJeune, as NOK.

She served in Halifax at the MD 6 Training Depot and CMH until falling ill in November 1918 and was SOS in February 1919. She was nursing at the Vincent Memorial Hospital in Boston in 1923.[242]

154. Leslie, Arthur Wilbert (1886–1936). Born in East Lawrencetown, Halifax County, s/o Adam (deceased) and Sarah (Gaetz) Leslie. He named his sister, Theresa, wife of Kester MacDonald, as NOK. He was a trained nurse working at the Nova Scotia Hospital when he joined the CEF as an orderly in the CAMC in August 1918. He served in MD 6 until being SOS in April 1919, then resumed nursing at the Nova Scotia Hospital.[243] He married Dorothy Brown in 1920, and they lived in Wilmot Station, Annapolis County.

155. Lester, Olla Dell (1892[244]–1958). Born in Truro, Colchester County, d/o Thomas and Mary (Baird) Lester, she was nursing in Halifax and had three months' CAMC experience when she joined the CAMCNS in October 1918. She served with the MD 6 Training Depot and as assistant director of medical services staff at CHH and subsidiaries until being SOS in July 1919. In 1923 she was nursing in Truro, Colchester County.[245] In 1927 she married Gerald Decourcey Hare, whose family had moved from Dartmouth to Edmonton, and worked there in the VON until 1931, when she retired.[246] Her brother, Robert Gordon Lester, enlisted in the 17th Battalion in 1914 but served overseas with the 1st Divisional Signal Company and was awarded the Military Medal "for extraordinary gallantry & devotion to duty & utter contempt for his personal safety" at Pozières in October 1916.

156. Logan, Carolyn "Carrie" Annette (1896–1956). Born in Little River, Halifax County, d/o Captain John and Mary (Wardrope) Logan, she was a graduate of Milford Hospital in Milford, Massachusetts, and had CAMC experience when she joined the CAMCNS in April 1918. She served at the MD 6 Training Depot and CHH and subsidiaries until being SOS in June 1919. She married Albert Garfield Wicks, who was a dental surgeon in Boston when he joined the CAMC with the rank of lieutenant, later captain, in Halifax in May 1918 and served there. They subsequently moved to Pittsburgh, Pennsylvania.

157. Lombard, Marie "Celeste." *See* Macdonell, Marie Celeste.

158. Lordly, Edwina Ratcliffe (1890–1981). Born in Chester, Lunenburg County, d/o Edwin and Evelina (Ratcliffe) Lordly, she was a trained nurse, claiming to have CAMC experience, and was living in London, England, when she joined the CAMCNS. She served in No. 2 CGH at Le Tréport in April 1915 and the DCRC in December 1915 but was granted sick leave through much of 1916 because of appendicitis and neurasthenia. She then transferred to Halifax for three months but returned to England in March 1917 and served in No. 3 CCCS and No. 7 CGH. She resigned in February 1918 to marry John Adrian Chamier, the son of Major General F. E. A. Chamier, who had

joined the Royal Flying Corps and rose to command the 15th Wing during the war. He subsequently played a major role in the technical evolution of the RAF between the two world wars, commanding the Air Defence Cadet Corps, which became the Air Training Corps in 1941, for which he was appointed air commodore and was knighted. She became a competitive alpine skier and participated in the 1936 Garmisch-Partenkirchen Winter Games. Their son, Patrick Chamier, also joined the RAF and died on active service in Zimbabwe in 1940. After John's death in 1974, Edwina retired in the village of Sway in Hampshire, England.

159. Lynch, Mary Theresa (1880–1949). Born in Halifax, Halifax County, d/o Dennis and Mary (MacAdam) Lynch, she was a 1908 graduate of the VGH School of Nursing and had CAMC experience when she shaved four years from her date of birth and joined the CAMCNS in December 1916. She served in No. 2 CGH, No. 4 CCCS, No. 16 CGH and No. 3 CGH until contracting influenza. She was mentioned in dispatches and received the Queen Elisabeth Medal (Belgium). She returned to Halifax in April 1919, reverted to the CAMC, and served in CHH and CMH until being demobilized in June 1920. In 1923 she married James Wall (*See* #299), a male nurse who served in No. 9 CSH as an orderly but later became a butcher, and they lived in Antigonish. *See* Wall, James.

160. Macaulay, Lorinda (1882–1951). Born in River John, Pictou County, d/o Alexander and Annie (Graham) Macaulay, Seafoam, Pictou County, she was a graduate of St. Joseph's Hospital School of Nursing. She joined the CAMCNS in October 1915 and served in No. 7 CGH until February 1916 when she contracted neurasthenia. Following treatment at the Canadian Convalescent Hospital at Bear Wood, Wokingham, Berkshire, she returned to Halifax on the *Llandovery Castle*'s last journey to Halifax in June 1918. She served in the MD 6 Training Depot, CMH and CHH until being demobilized in March 1920. She returned home and was nursing at Tatamagouche, Colchester County, when she died.

161. MacCuish, Elizabeth Margaret (1891–1968). Born in Sydney Mines, Cape Breton, d/o John (deceased) and Mary Jane (MacDonald) MacCuish, and sister of Harriet Mary (MacCuish) MacKinnon, she was a 1916 graduate of the VGH School of Nursing and had sixteen months' CAMC experience when she joined the CAMCNS in December 1917. She served in No. 14 CGH, No. 13 CGH, No. 3 CSH and No. 8 CSH until being SOS in April 1919. In 1923 she was nursing at Harbourview Hospital in Sydney Mines.[247] In 1924 she married Kenneth MacDonald, a miner, and they moved to Everett, and later Somerville, Massachusetts.

162. MacCuish, Harriet Mary. *See* MacKinnon, Harriet Mary.

163. MacDonald, Annie (1875–1959). Born in Sydney Mines, Cape Breton, d/o Kenneth and Euphemia (McKinnon) MacDonald and wife of Albert House, she shaved three years from her date of birth when she joined the CAMC-NS in April 1916. She served in the DCRC, No. 9 CSH and No. 7 CGH, then was transferred to Halifax, reverted to the CAMC and served at CHH and CMH until being SOS in March 1920. She, her husband and two children were living in Sydney Mines in 1921.

164. MacDonald, Annie Belle (1887–?) Born in Antigonish, Antigonish County, d/o John B. and Flora (MacDonald) MacDonald, Glassburn, Antigonish County, she was nursing in Montreal when she joined the CAMCNS in February 1916 and served in No. 6 CGH (Laval), the Moore Barracks Hospital at Shorncliffe, No. 8 CGH, No. 2 CGH and No. 7 CGH until being transferred to Halifax where she reverted to the CAMC and served in CHH and subsidiaries until being SOS in January 1920. Her brother, Daniel MacDonald, became a priest, joined the faculty of St. Francis Xavier University in 1912, and was president from 1936 to 1944.

165. MacDonald, Annie Helen (1890–1955). Born in Ardness, Pictou County, d/o Hugh and Margaret (McNeil) MacDonald, she joined the CAMCNS in April 1916 and served in No. 9 CSH, the Granville Canadian Special Hospital, No. 12 CGH, No. 7 CGH and No. 3 CSH until being SOS in August 1919. In 1920 she married Alexander Lauchlin MacNeill, a farmer from Harbour Centre, Antigonish County, who had enlisted in the 193rd Battalion in March 1916 but served as a sergeant in the 85th Battalion and was wounded.

166. MacDonald, Catherine Chisholm (1879–1959). Born in Heatherton, Antigonish County, d/o Angus (deceased) and Annie (Chisholm) MacDonald, she joined the CAMCNS at Antigonish in April 1916. She served in No. 9 CSH and the Canadian Convalescent Officers' Hospital at Matlock Bath, then returned to Halifax in October in 1918, reverted to the CAMC, and nursed at CHH until being SOS in October 1919. She then resumed nursing in Antigonish.

167. MacDonald, Catherine Eileen (1888–1970). Born in Arisaig, Antigonish County, d/o John Angus (deceased) and Annie MacDonald, she joined the CAMCNS in April 1916 and served in No. 9 CSH, the Moore Barracks Hospital at Shorncliffe, later designated No. 11 CGH, and No. 7 CGH. She returned to Halifax in August 1919, reverted to the CAMC, and served at CHH from August 1919 until demobilization in January 1920. She continued nursing in Halifax until retiring in 1955.

168. MacDonald, Catherine Tulloch (1870–1959). Born in Brook Village, Inverness County, d/o Alexander and Margaret (MacDonald) MacDonald, she was nursing in Halifax and had four months' CAMC experience with No.

8 Field Ambulance when she shaved ten years from her date of birth and joined the CAMCNS in May 1916. She served in the Granville Canadian Special Hospital, No. 2 CGH, No. 9 CSH, No. 3 CGH, No. 4 CGH and No. 15 CGH. In May 1919 she was transferred to Halifax, reverted to the CAMC, and served in CHH until being SOS in June 1919. She was living in Brook Village in 1924–25[248] but also nursed in Halifax until retiring in 1944.

169. MacDonald, Evaline "Eva" May (1894–1972). Born in West River Station, Pictou County, d/o William Angus and Catherine (Bruce) MacDonald, Abercrombie, Pictou County, she studied nursing in New York or Baltimore and served in the American Ambulance Hospital, established in 1914 at Neuilly, attached to the American Hospital of Paris but under the French Service de Santé des Armées. The physicians and nurses were recruited from the Presbyterian and St. Luke's Hospitals in New York and Johns Hopkins Hospital in Baltimore. The American Red Cross took it over in 1917 and renamed it Red Cross Hospital No. 1. In 1920 she married George Matheson, a farmer at Lansdowne, Pictou County.

170. Macdonald, Evangeline "Eva" (1889–1966). Born in Iron Rock, Pictou County, d/o Hugh (deceased) and Mary (Cameron) Macdonald, Bridgeville, Pictou County, she studied maternity nursing at the Wesson Maternity Hospital in Springhill, Massachusetts,[249] and was a 1914 graduate of the VGH School of Nursing. She was nursing in Halifax with twenty-eight months' CAMC experience when she joined the CAMCNS in July 1918. She served at the CMH, CHH and Camp Aldershot until being SOS in January 1919. She married Alfred Haliburton, descendant of T. C. Haliburton, lawyer, judge, politician, and author of *The Clockmaker: or, the Sayings and Doings of Samuel Slick, of Slickville*, first published by Joseph Howe in 1836. Alfred was a Halifax banker who served as a captain with the MD 6 Royal Canadian Garrison Artillery in the war. Following her husband's death in a motor vehicle accident in 1925, she resumed private nursing.[250] Their three sons served in the Second World War, and one, William Haliburton, served as a pilot in the RCAF and was killed in May 1942, making Eva a Silver Cross Mother.

171. Macdonald, Georgina Emily (1882–?). Born in Pictou, Pictou County, d/o Allan and Elizabeth (MacLean) Macdonald, she was nursing in Halifax and had CAMC experience when she joined the CAMCNS in April 1917. She served in England in the Kitchener Military Hospital (redesignated No. 10 CGH in September 1917), the CAMC Casualty Company and No. 16 CGH until returning to Halifax and being SOS in March 1919.

172. MacDonald, Harriett Helena (1888–1969). Born in Trenton, Pictou County, d/o James and Isabella (Powell) MacDonald, she was nursing in Halifax

and had eight months' CAMC experience when she joined the CAMCNS in July 1918. She served in the MD 6 Training Depot, the Prince Edward Island Military Convalescent Hospital and CHH until being SOS in May 1919. She moved to Sydney, Cape Breton County, in 1944,[251] probably because her sister was living there, and continued nursing until 1949.

173. MacDonald, Harriett "Hilda" (1891–1976). Born in Sydney, Cape Breton, d/o Angus (deceased) and Harriett (Moorhouse) MacDonald, she may have studied nursing at McGill University because she joined the CAMCNS in Montreal in April 1915. She served in No. 3 CGH (McGill) in Montreal, RAMC No. 6 Military Hospital at Shorncliffe, No. 2 CCCS, No. 10 CGH and No. 9 CGH until being SOS in May 1919. While in London, she appears to have met Major William Macintosh, a Scottish artilleryman, whose family had emigrated from Scotland to Winnipeg in 1903, then to Saskatoon, and when they returned to Canada in 1919, they married.[252] Their son Angus Macintosh served in the Royal Canadian Artillery in the Second World War and was killed in September 1944.

174. MacDonald, Helen Catherine (1888–1965). Born in Little Narrows, Victoria County, d/o John (deceased) and Jessie Catherine (Maclean) MacDonald, she was nursing in Halifax and had CAMC experience when she joined the CAMCNS in December 1916. She named her mother, who was living in Sydney, Cape Breton County, as her NOK. She served in No. 1 CGH, No. 9 CGH and No. 14 CGH until returning to Halifax in June 1919 and being SOS in November 1919. She was still nursing in Sydney in 1949 but moved to San Jose, California, where she married Edward Klein, who had served in the US Army in France. They later moved to Santa Clara, where she died in 1965.[253]

175. MacDonald, Hilda Havergal (1885–1990). Born in Glendyer, Inverness County, d/o Walter and Annabel (Cameron) MacDonald (both deceased), she was a 1913 graduate of the Presbyterian Hospital (now Columbia University Hospital) School of Nursing in New York. She joined the CAMCNS in September 1915, naming her sister, Hannah Macdonald, as her NOK. She served in the DCRC, No. 2 CGH at Le Tréport, the CAMC Training School and the Moore Barracks Hospital at Shorncliffe, later designated No. 11 CGH, then returned to France with No. 3 CCCS and was awarded the Royal Red Cross 2nd Class. She also served in No. 2 CGH, the King's Canadian Red Cross Special Hospital at Bushy Park, the IODE Hospital in London and the Canadian Convalescent Officers' Hospital at Matlock Bath until returning to Canada in March 1919. She was temporarily posted to nursing services in Ottawa until being SOS in August 1919. She nursed for four years in Saskatchewan, then at the Nova Scotia Teachers College in Truro until retiring in Wolfville and Glendyer.

176. Macdonald, Janet McGregor (1892–1968). Born in Big Island, Pictou County, d/o James and Isabelle (McGregor) Macdonald, and a cousin of Margaret Clotilde Macdonald. She joined the CAMCNS in Quebec City in September 1914, naming her father as NOK, and served in the Canadian Convalescent Hospital in London, No. 16 CGH, No. 10 CSH, No. 1 CCCS and No. 2 CGH, of which she was acting matron with the rank of captain. She was awarded the 1914 Star, both the Royal Red Cross 2nd Class and the Royal Red Cross 1st Class and was mentioned in dispatches. When she returned to Canada in September 1919, she was posted to Ste. Anne's Military Hospital in Montreal until being SOS in January 1920. She resumed nursing in Montreal and in 1925 married William Smith Beattie, a British bank manager, who lived in Mexico City until he moved to Montreal in 1932.[254]
177. MacDonald, Jessie (1880–1937). Born in Copper Lake, Antigonish County, d/o Murdoch and Mary (Kennedy) MacDonald, she was a 1915 graduate of the VGH School of Nursing and joined the CAMCNS in April 1916. She served in No. 9 CSH, the Canadian Convalescent Hospital at Uxbridge, and the Moore Barracks Hospital at Shorncliffe (later designated No. 11 CGH). When she developed health issues in July 1917, she was attached to HMHS *Letitia*, which carried convalescent soldiers to Halifax, and was allowed to resign from the CAMCNS in August 1917. She was then appointed head nurse in the VGH operating room and was there when the Halifax Explosion took place.[255] In October 1921 she retired and returned to Copper Lake. She continued nursing in Antigonish until retiring in 1935 and dying there.[256] Her nephew, Roderick MacDonald, served in the Royal Navy Air Service and the Royal Air Force and was killed in May 1918.
178. MacDonald, Jessie Helen (1882–1973). Born in Coalburn, Pictou County, d/o John and Margaret (MacIntosh) MacDonald, New Glasgow, Pictou County, she was a 1915 graduate of the VGH School of Nursing and was the head nurse in the VGH operating room when she shaved four years off her date of birth and joined the CAMCNS in March 1917. She served in No. 7 CSH, the Shorncliffe Military Hospital, No. 9 CGH, No. 6 CGH, the CAMC Casualty Company, and No. 15 CGH until returning home. She reverted to the CAMC and served briefly in CHH before being SOS in July 1919. She returned to Coalburn and continued nursing in New Glasgow until retiring in 1952.[257]
179. MacDonald, Louise Agnes (1883–1964). Born in Salt Springs, Antigonish County, d/o Angus and Margaret (Fuller) MacDonald, she was nursing in Montreal and had CAMC experience when she joined the CAMCNS in June 1915. She served in the Moore Barracks Hospital at Shorncliffe (later designated No. 11 CGH), No. 2 CGH, No. 3 CGH at Le Tréport, No. 1 CCCS, and No. 12 CGH and was awarded the Royal Red Cross 2nd Class.

In June 1919 she reverted to the CAMC and served in CHH until being SOS in January 1920. She returned to Antigonish and nursed there until her retirement. Her father taught at St. Francis Xavier University, was appointed school inspector for Antigonish and Guysborough Counties, and then taught mathematics at the Provincial Normal School and served as mayor in 1907–8 and 1915–16. Two of her brothers served in the war. Angus Macdonald enlisted in the 225th Battalion in September 1916 but served in the 54th Battalion and was killed at Lens in September 1917. William Gladstone Macdonald served as a lieutenant in the 85th Battalion.

180. MacDonald, Margaret (1884–?). Born in Glace Bay, Cape Breton, she was a graduate of the St. Joseph's Hospital School of Nursing in Glace Bay and listed her brother, Michael MacDonald, Sydney, as her NOK when she joined the CAMCNS in October 1915. She served in No. 7 CSH, was mentioned in dispatches in May 1918, and was awarded the Royal Red Cross 2nd Class, then served briefly with the Canadian Forestry Corps Hospital at Lajoux and the CAMC Casualty Company at Shorncliffe before being transferred to Halifax in June 1919. She served in CHH and CMH until being SOS in February 1920 and served as matron of the Sydney Marine Hospital until returning to Glace Bay.

181. Macdonald, Margaret[258] Clotilde (1873–1948). Born in Baileys Brook, Pictou County, d/o Donald (deceased) and Mary Elizabeth (Chisholm) Macdonald, and cousin of Janet McGregor Macdonald,[259] she was an 1895 graduate of the Charity Hospital School for Nurses in New York City, then served as a nurse in Panama during the construction of the canal and nursed American soldiers during the Spanish-American War.[260] She also served as a nurse in the South African War and joined the CAMC in 1906. When the First World War broke out in 1914, she was appointed matron-in-chief of the CAMCNS with the rank of major, responsible for all Canadian military nurses serving overseas, despite shaving six years from her date of birth. She was awarded the Royal Red Cross 1st Class, the Florence Nightingale Medal and an honorary degree from St. Francis Xavier University. Indeed, according to Allan Marble, she was the most decorated nursing sister among the Allied Forces.[261] She retired in 1923 and in 1926 unveiled the memorial to Canada's nursing sisters in the parliament building. In 1983 she was posthumously recognized as a person of national historic significance with a plaque at Baileys Brook.

182. Macdonald, Margaret Katherine (1885–1971). Born in Thorburn, Pictou County, d/o Evan (deceased) and Ellen (McDonald) Macdonald, she may have trained in Massachusetts, then moved to Halifax and was nursing there. She had sixteen months' CAMC experience when she joined the

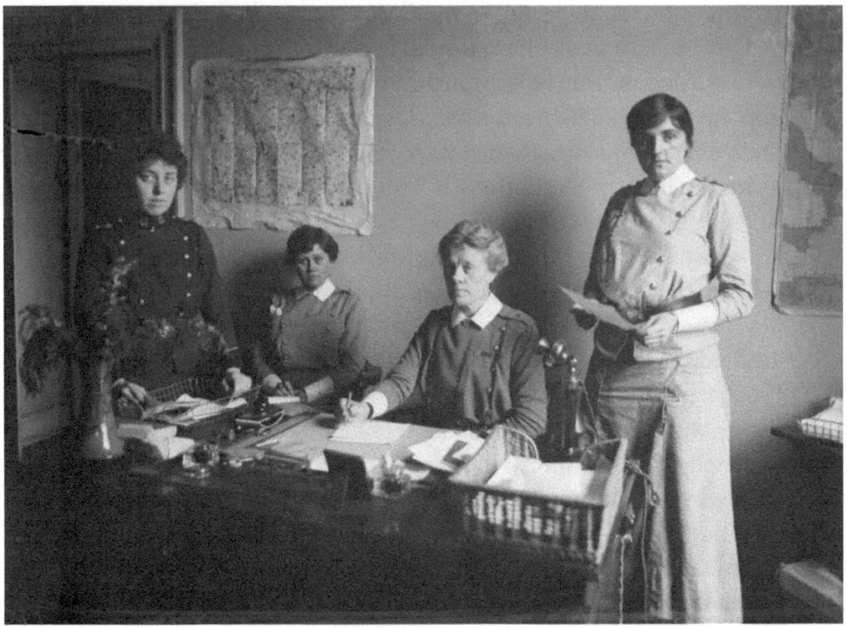

Margaret Clotilde Macdonald (*See* #181).
[CANADA, DEPT. OF NATIONAL DEFENCE/LIBRARY AND ARCHIVES CANADA]

CAMCNS in July 1918. She served in the MD 6 Training Depot and CHH until being SOS in May 1919. In 1920 she was nursing in Chicago, then back in Thorburn in 1923–24, but by 1930 was a hotel nurse in Cambridge, Massachusetts. She settled in Lowell, Massachusetts, and when she died, she was buried in the Edson Cemetery there.[262]

183. MacDonald, Mary Margaret (1877–1955). Born in Hopewell, Pictou County, d/o Enon and Isabella MacDonald, she was a 1911 graduate of the VGH School of Nursing and shaved six years off her age when she joined the CAMCNS in December 1915. She served in No. 7 CSH and No. 12 CGH until May 1918 when she returned to Halifax and served in CHH and CMH until being SOS in March 1920. She lived in Hopewell but did not continue nursing.

184. MacDonald, Mary "Minnie" Frances (1889–1984). Born in New Glasgow, Pictou County, d/o John and Mary (McDonald) MacDonald, she was a graduate of St. Joseph's Hospital School of Nursing and was living in New Glasgow when she joined the CAMCNS in April 1916, naming her father as NOK. She served in No. 9 CSH, No. 1 CGH, No. 4 CGH, and No. 2 CGH when it was bombed, then No. 16 CGH. She returned to Halifax in July 1919,

reverted to the CAMC, and served at CHH until demobilization in January 1920. She served as night nursing supervisor in a hospital in Greenville, South Carolina, until returning home, and in 1927 married John Ambrose McLeod. Born in Reserve Mines, Cape Breton, he was a clerk, living in nearby McKays Corner when he joined No. 9 CSH in Antigonish in 1916 and was promoted to sergeant major, then to warrant officer in 1917. He later worked for the Dominion Coal Company and died in 1961.

185. MacDonald, Mary Simpson (1892–1962). Born in Baddeck, Victoria County, d/o Alexander and Alice (Crowdis) MacDonald, she was a 1911 graduate of the Friends Hospital School of Nursing in Philadelphia and had brief CAMC experience at the CMH when she joined the CAMCNS in May 1917. She served in the DCRC, No. 10 CSH, No. 3 CSH and No. 15 CGH, then returned to Halifax in July 1919 and served in CHH and the CMH until being SOS in March 1920. She married George Farnsworth, who was born in Digby, Digby County, but was living in Charlestown, Massachusetts, when he enlisted in the CEF in Montreal in November 1917 and did not serve overseas. They married in Philadelphia, Pennsylvania, in 1921, but moved to Detroit, Michigan, and died there.

186. Macdonell, Marie Celeste (1887–1976). Born in Little Brook, Digby County, d/o Jean (deceased) and Marguerite (Leblanc) Lombard, she married Dr. Winfred Smythe Macdonell, Port Hood, Inverness, in 1914. She was a 1911 graduate of the VGH School of Nursing and was nursing at the VGH when she went to England in 1915. There she joined the QAIMNS and served in the Queen Alexandra Military Hospital in London before transferring into the CAMCNS in August 1915. She served briefly in the DCRC, No. 2 CGH and the Canadian Convalescent Hospital at Uxbridge. Her husband went to London in September 1916 and joined the CAMC with the rank of captain, then acting major. When he died of pneumonia in London in November 1918, she resigned and settled in Sydney, Cape Breton County, where she worked as a school nurse.[263]

187. MacDougald, Margaret[264] (1888–?). Born in Antigonish, Antigonish County, d/o Ronald and Mary (Malloy) Macdougald, she appears to have trained in Montreal and was nursing there when she joined No. 6 CGH at Laval in January 1916, naming her sister, Mrs. H. MacDonald, as NOK. She also served in the Moore Barracks Hospital at Shorncliffe (later designated No. 11 CGH), No. 8 CGH, No. 2 CGH, the Westcliffe Canadian Eye and Ear Hospital and the CAMC Casualty Company. In February 1919 she was transferred to Halifax and served in CHH until being SOS in May 1919. In 1965 she moved to Knoydart, a rural coastal community on the Sunrise Trail between Lismore and the eastern boundary between Antigonish and Pictou Counties.

188. MacDougall, Flora (1880–1957). Born in Cape George, Antigonish County, d/o Archibald and Annie (MacDonald) Macdougall, she studied nursing in Massachusetts and was a public health nurse in Boston before joining her family in Maryvale, Antigonish County. In April 1916 she joined the CAMCNS and served in No. 9 CSH, No. 1 CGH, No. 10 CSH and the CAMC Casualty Company until being transferred to Halifax in July 1919. Then she reverted to the CAMC and served at CHH and subsidiaries until being SOS in January 1920. She continued nursing at CHH until 1924, when she was appointed public health nurse of Antigonish County. She retired in 1928, when the Sisters of St. Martha took charge of public health work for the county.[265] In later years she lived in Halifax but returned to Maryvale and died there.[266]

189. MacInnes, Ellaphallie Curry (1892–1949). Born in Halifax, Halifax County, d/o Ronald (deceased) and Carrie (McHeffey) MacInnes. She had two years' CAMC experience when she joined the CAMCNS in November 1918. She served in Halifax in the CMH until being SOS in April 1919. She moved to Virden, Manitoba, in 1921 and married Lyle Simpson, who lived in Brandon and had joined the 79th Battalion in 1915 but served in the 10th Battalion. They presumably met when he was demobilized in Halifax in 1919, and they lived in New Westminster, British Columbia.

190. MacInnes, Florence Louisa (1881–1969). Born in Halifax, Halifax County, d/o Henry (deceased) and Frances (Gladwin) MacInnes. She was a 1909 graduate of the VGH School of Nursing and was night supervisor at the VGH from 1911 to 1913 and later assistant superintendent of nurses. She had two months' CAMC experience at the CMH when she joined the CAMCNS in London in May 1915. While serving in No. 1 CGH at Étaples from May to August 1916, she and the other nurses experienced air raids and were "constantly exposed to horrific injuries and long periods of overwork with no rest" and again in April 1917, when a German airplane bombed the area, resulting in her being admitted to Granville Canadian Special Hospital, Ramsgate, which treated shellshock and other nervous diseases. A month later she was transferred to the Westcliffe Nursing Sisters' Home in Margate, then was returned to Canada for further medical treatment at Montreal and later Pine Hill Convalescent Hospital in Halifax in July 1919. She ceased nursing and worked in local businesses until retiring in the late 1940s.[267]

191. MacInnis, Dorothea Jeanne (1887–1962). Born in Hillside Mira, Cape Breton, d/o Donald and Anna (McLennan) MacInnis. She studied nursing in the United States, had served in the QAIMNS and had sixteen months' experience in the Harvard Surgical Unit with RAMC No. 22 General Hospital at

Étaples when she transferred into the CAMCNS in London in March 1918. She served in No. 10 CGH until March 1919 when she was SOS and returned to Halifax. She was living with her family in 1921 but moved to Gloucester, Massachusetts, where she nursed in the Addison Gilbert Hospital. In 1925 she married George Cardno Edward, a sea captain, and they lived in Belmont, Massachusetts. He served in the Australian Merchant Navy in the Second World War and died in 1943 when his ship, SS *Fort Longueuil*, was sunk by a submarine.[268]

192. MacIntosh, Mary Catherine (1885–1974). Born in St. Andrews, Antigonish County, d/o Duncan (deceased) and Margaret (Chisholm) MacIntosh, Lower South River, Antigonish County, she joined the CAMCNS in Montreal in April 1916. She served in the DCRC, No. 4 CGH and No. 5 CGH but fell ill at Salonika in April 1917 and returned to England. She served in No. 4 CGH at Basingstoke, No. 8 CSH and No. 3 CGH until returning to Halifax and was SOS in July 1919. In 1920 she married Maurice Lynch, a federal civil servant who lived in Almonte, Ontario, whose father, Dr. John Lynch, was the physician of the Dominion Iron and Steel Company in Sydney. Maurice had three months' experience with the CMH, presumably as an orderly, when he joined the CAMC in Halifax in November 1914. He attended the CAMC Training School at Shorncliffe near Cheriton, Kent, then served in No. 1 CGH, the DCRC, No. 4 Company, Canadian Forestry Corps, and No. 5 Field Ambulance with the rank of sergeant. They lived in Ottawa.

193. MacIntosh, Rebecca (1892–1917). Born in Pleasant Bay, Inverness County, d/o Peter (deceased) and Eliza "Christy" (Sutherland) MacIntosh. She was a 1915 graduate of the VGH School of Nursing. She was living with her mother and nursing in Truro when she joined the CAMCNS in Halifax in April 1917, naming her brother, Rev. John Peter McIntosh, as NOK. She served in No. 10 CGH at Brighton until December 1918 when she was transferred to No. 9 CGH at Kinmel Park in Wales, a transit camp for Canadian soldiers waiting for transport home. When influenza ravaged the camp in March 1919, she died and was buried in nearby St. Margaret's Cemetery at Bodelwyddan, alongside 208 Canadian soldiers, most of whom also died of influenza. Her brother died of influenza a month later. She was commemorated on both the Pleasant Bay and Truro cenotaphs and the Celtic Cross at St. Matthew's United Church in Halifax. She was also commemorated on the memorial to overseas nurses who died in the war in the nurses' residence at the Elizabeth Garrett Women's Hospital in London, but it has since been demolished.

194. MacIsaac, Sarah Catherine (1882–1969). Born in Arisaig, Antigonish County, d/o John and Mary (MacDonald) MacIsaac, she was a graduate of Mount

Saint Bernard College in Antigonish and St. Joseph's Hospital and was head nurse of its operating room for three years. She then completed postgraduate training at Mercy Hospital in Chicago and was assistant matron at Mount Zion Hospital in San Francisco when she returned to Antigonish and joined the CAMCNS in March 1916 as matron of No. 9 CSH. When it was bombed in a German air raid in May 1916, killing two medical staff, one of whom was Horace Goddard MacMillan of Isaacs Harbour, Guysborough County, she was mentioned in dispatches and was awarded the Royal Red Cross 2nd Class and the Royal Red Cross 1st Class. She returned to England in May 1919, then was transferred to Halifax and served as matron of CHH until being SOS in July 1919. She continued nursing there until retiring in 1947.

195. Mack, Beatrice Helena (1883–1928). Born in Mill Village, Queens County, d/o Isaac Newton and Rachel (Vaughan) Mack, Liverpool, Queens County, she was a 1906 graduate of the Women's Charity Club Hospital in Brookline, Massachusetts, and had CAMC experience when she joined the CAMCNS in Halifax in April 1915. She served in the DCRC, No. 11 CSH, No. 1 CGH, No. 16 CGH, the Canadian Officers' Hospital in London, the Canadian Red Cross Officers Hospital and No. 15 CGH until contracting diphtheria. She returned to Halifax and was demobilized in March 1919. She was living in Liverpool, Queens County, in 1921 but in 1923 married Aimé Joseph Gieger in Pepperell, Massachusetts, and died in 1928 in Nashua, New Hampshire.[269] Her father was a merchant who briefly represented Queens County in the Nova Scotia Assembly from 1874 to 1878 and was its speaker in 1877–78.

196. MacKenzie, Charlotte (1888–1993). Born in Leitches Creek, Cape Breton, d/o Daniel and Christine (Fraser) MacKenzie, she may have trained at McGill or Laval because she was nursing in Montreal when she joined No. 6 CSH (Laval) in December 1915. She also served at the Moore Barracks Hospital (later designated No. 11 CGH), No. 2 CGH, the Shorncliffe CAMC Depot and No. 11 CGH until being transferred to Halifax and was SOS in April 1919. She was nursing in Sackville, New Brunswick, in 1921 but two years later moved to the United States and in 1925 married Jonathan Livingston, who was from New Brunswick but lived in Putnam, New York. They subsequently lived in Framingham, Massachusetts, and Stoddard, New Hampshire, but she later returned to Sydney Mines.

197. MacKenzie, Christina Mary (1881–1967). Born in Lower Middle River, Victoria County, d/o Christopher (deceased) and Annie (MacDonald) MacKenzie and sister of Margaret Eliza MacKenzie and Minnie Hannah MacKenzie, she had CAMC experience when she joined the CAMCNS in May 1916. She served in No. 9 CSH, No. 3 CSH and No. 11 CGH until being transferred in

June 1919 to Halifax, where she served in CHH and CMH and was SOS in March 1920. She continued nursing in Halifax and retired there.

198. MacKenzie, Dora (1886–1959). Born at Joggins Mines, Cumberland County, d/o John and Mary Ann (Devine) (deceased) MacKenzie. She joined the CAMCNS in April 1916 and served in No. 9 CSH, No. 12 CGH and No. 16 CGH, then returned to Halifax and was SOS in August 1919. She later moved to North Branford, Connecticut, but may have lived in Montrose, Pennsylvania, where her brother Garfield MacKenzie and his family lived, years later, because she was buried there.

199. Mackenzie, Edith Mary (1883–1964). Born in Halifax, Halifax County, d/o William and Catherine (Beamish) Mackenzie, she was a 1908 graduate of the VGH School of Nursing and had CAMC experience in the CMH when she joined the CAMCNS in December 1916. She served in the Shorncliffe Military Hospital, the Shorncliffe CAMC Depot, No. 2 CGH, No. 14 CGH, No. 9 CGH, the CAMC Casualty Company, the DCRC and No. 11 CGH but had health problems and returned to Halifax and was SOS in September 1919. She later moved to Weston, Ontario, where she married William Thomas Hall, a Toronto salesman who had served in the 3rd Battalion, was wounded three times, promoted to lieutenant, and was awarded the Distinguished Conduct Medal in January 1919.

200. MacKenzie, Helen Gertrude (1863–1954). Born in Pictou, Pictou County, d/o George and Catherine (Fogo) MacKenzie, she had nearly three years' CAMC experience nursing at the Moxham Castle and Ross Military Convalescent Hospitals in Sydney when, despite being fifty-five years old, she joined the CAMCNS in November 1918, naming her brother, George MacKenzie, as NOK. After being SOS in January 1919, she lived in Stellarton, Pictou County, in 1923 and then Halifax.

201. MacKenzie, Margaret Eliza (1883–1969). Born in Lower Middle River, Victoria County, d/o Christopher (deceased) and Ann (MacDonald) MacKenzie, Halifax, and sister of Christina Mary MacKenzie and Minnie Hannah MacKenzie. She was a 1908 graduate of the VGH School of Nursing and was night supervisor of nurses until 1910, then superintendent of nurses in All Saints Hospital in Springhill, Cumberland County. In September 1915 she shaved two years from her date of birth and joined the CAMCNS in London. She served in No. 3 CSH at Lemnos and Salonika, No. 7 CGH, No. 2 CSH, King's Canadian Red Cross Special Hospital and No. 16 CGH but developed serious health issues and was invalided to Halifax in June 1919. She subsequently undertook postgraduate studies in social service at the University of Toronto and was appointed the first director of Nova Scotia's Department of Public Health in 1920. She served as president of

the RNANS in 1930–32. When she retired to Montreal in 1954, the Canadian Public Health Association awarded her emerita status for outstanding service in the field of public health. She later returned to Halifax. In 2009 the College of Registered Nurses of Nova Scotia awarded her the Centennial Award of Distinction posthumously for her contribution to nursing.

202. MacKenzie, Minnie Hannah (1888–1972). Born in Lower Middle River, Victoria County, d/o Christopher (deceased) and Annie (MacDonald) MacKenzie, Halifax, and sister of Christina Mary MacKenzie and Margaret Eliza MacKenzie. She joined the CAMCNS at Halifax in April 1917 and served in the Kitchener Military Hospital (redesignated No. 10 CGH in September 1917) and the CAMC Casualty Company. She fell seriously ill in November 1918, was transferred to Halifax in January 1919 and was SOS in May 1919. She later lived in Toronto and in 1938 married Athol Mayhew, son of Henry Mayhew, a prominent British writer, who had emigrated to Canada and was a widower. Athol served as a lieutenant in the 35th Battalion but was SOS in 1917 because of illness. His son from the first marriage, Jerrold Mayhew, was killed in the Canadian raid on Dieppe in 1943. After Athol's death in 1945, Minnie moved to Greenville, South Carolina, and applied for social security in 1966.

203. MacKinnon, Alice. *See* Blood, Alice.

204. MacKinnon, Harriet Mary (1890–1972). Born in Whycocomagh, Inverness County, d/o John (deceased) and Mary Jane (MacDonald) MacKinnon and sister of Elizabeth Margaret MacCuish. She was a 1910 graduate of the St. Joseph's Hospital School of Nursing and the wife of Dr. Kenneth MacCuish of St. Peters, Richmond County. He taught at St. Joseph's and practised in Glace Bay with Dr. Angus MacLeod before joining No. 9 Field Ambulance and was killed at Passchendaele in October 1917. She moved to Halifax and lived with another sister, Mary MacCuish. She had six weeks' CAMC experience when she joined the CAMCNS in August 1918, naming Mary her NOK. She served in No. 12 CGH in England and the MD 6 Training Depot until being SOS in August 1919. She nursed in Sydney until 1960 and retired to Baddeck, Victoria County, in about 1966.

205. MacKinnon, Ruth (1894–1978). Born in New Glasgow, Pictou County, d/o Charles and Mary Jane (Ross) MacKinnon, she was nursing in Halifax and had eighteen months' CAMC experience when she joined the CAMCNS in July 1918. She served in Halifax at the MD 6 Training Depot and the CMH until being SOS in May 1919. She moved to Boston in 1920 and married Edward Sullivan, who served in the US army, and they moved to Santa Clara, California. After his death in 1943, she lived with their daughter, Margaret, and her family in Arlington, Massachusetts.

206. MacLatchy, Katherine Osborne (1874–1969). Born in Grand Pré, Kings County, d/o Edward and Sophia (Borden) MacLatchy and a niece of Robert Borden. She was a graduate of the Montreal (McGill) General Hospital School of Nursing and joined the CAMCNS in May 1915 as matron of No. 3 (McGill) CGH, naming her brother, Arthur MacLatchy, as NOK. She was awarded the Royal Red Cross 1st Class in October 1917, then was transferred to Halifax in May 1919 and served as principal matron for MD 6, responsible for both CHH and CMH, until being SOS in June 1920. She continued nursing at CHH until retiring to Grand Pré in 1930. She was one of the founders of the GNANS and played a major role in its replacement in 1922 by the Registered Nurses' Association of Nova Scotia (RNANS), which introduced the RN designation.

207. MacLean, Catherine (1875–1943). Born in Sydney Mines, Cape Breton, d/o Hector (deceased) and Sarah (MacLean) MacLean, she was a 1904 graduate of the VGH School of Nursing and joined the CAMCNS in October 1915 despite being over age, allegedly because of the death of her fiancé in Demerara, South America, but perhaps because her father had died in August. She served in No. 7 CSH until September 1917 when she was transferred to the Moxham Castle Convalescent Hospital in Sydney. She was SOS in March 1919 for health reasons, was treated at the Queen's Military Hospital in Kingston, Ontario, and recovered. She continued nursing in Sydney Mines. She took many photographs while overseas and also left an autograph book that includes the signatures of many soldiers.

208. MacLean, Elizabeth Isabella (1885–1973). Born in Big Island, Pictou County, d/o Rev. Lauchlin and Margaret (Thompson) MacLean and sister of Neil MacLean, Pictou, Pictou County, she was a 1910 graduate of the VGH School of Nursing and was an operating room nurse there. She had fourteen months' CAMC experience in Halifax, when she joined the CAMCNS in May 1917. She served with the DCRC and the CAMC Casualty Company, then was SOS and returned to Halifax in April 1919. She and three other nurses moved to Montreal and then to the Peace River area in northern Alberta in 1921 to take advantage of free land grants for veterans offered by the federal government. She soon discovered that her medical skills were needed in the community of Rycroft, and "never took a penny for her services."[270] In 1924 she married Louis Young, who had also settled in the area. In 1966 the community celebrated the official opening of the Elizabeth Young Municipal Park in her honour. Her three brothers served overseas in the CEF and were all killed in action. Despite being a trained nurse, Neil MacLean (*See* #212) served as a stretcher bearer in the 25th Battalion and died in action in September 1916. James and Hector served in the 85th Battalion and were killed in June 1917 and January 1918.

209. MacLean, Josephine (1886–1971). Born in Antigonish, Antigonish County, d/o James (deceased) and Anne (McDougall) MacLean, Glace Bay, she was nursing in Halifax and had two weeks' CAMC experience when she joined the CAMCNS in August 1918. She served in CHH from January to May 1919, then returned to Glace Bay.
210. MacLean, Marguerite (1891–?). Born in North Sydney, Cape Breton, d/o Dr. John and Ada (MacKeen) MacLean. She was the chief operating nurse at St. Luke's Hospital in Ottawa when she went to London in August 1915 and joined the CAMCNS. She served in the DCRC, No. 1 CGH, No. 2 CGH and No. 7 CGH until being transferred to MD 6 in February 1919 and was SOS in April 1919. She served briefly at the North Toronto Military Orthopedic Hospital, commonly referred to as the Davisville Hospital because it was situated on "Whiz-Bang Corner," the corner of Davisville Avenue and Yonge Street, then resumed nursing at St. Luke's Hospital. When it closed in 1924, she may have nursed at the Ottawa Civic Hospital and was still there in 1953. Her brother Isaac MacLean had four months' service in the Dalhousie University Canadian Officer's Training Corps (COTC) and enlisted in the University of Toronto COTC in September 1916 while a student there but transferred into the Royal Flying Corps in October 1916 and was wounded. In the Second World War he served as an RCAF squadron leader in Edmonton until dying in a flying accident in 1944. Another brother, Hector MacLean, who had moved to Manitoba, enlisted in September 1918 and joined the Royal North-West Mounted Police but died of influenza while training at Regina in October 1918.
211. MacLean, Mary Rachel (1887–1972). Born in Glace Bay, Cape Breton, d/o Donald and Christina "Christy" Ann (MacDonald) MacLean, she had CAMC experience when she shaved three years from her date of birth and joined the CAMCNS in Halifax in May 1917. She served in the DCRC, No. 15 CGH, No. 2 CSH, the CAMC Casualty Company and No. 9 CSH and was SOS in August 1919. She later nursed in Donkin and Glace Bay.
212. MacLean, Neil (1889–1916). Born in Big Island, Pictou County, s/o Rev. Lauchlin and Elizabeth (Thompson) MacLean and brother of Elizabeth MacLean, he had attended the Acadia Collegiate Academy, was a 1911 graduate of the VGH School of Nursing and had begun studying medicine in 1914 when he enlisted in the 25th Battalion in January 1915. Despite being a trained nurse, he served as a stretcher bearer with the rank of lance corporal. During the Battle of Courcelette in September 1915, he was promoted to medical orderly with the rank of sergeant but was one of some 450 men killed in action in the battle.[271] His two brothers, James Macglashan MacLean and Hector Norman MacLean, also served overseas

and were killed in June 1917 and January 1918. His sister, Elizabeth MacLean (*See* #208), had fourteen months' CAMC experience in Halifax when she joined the CAMCNS in May 1917.

213. Maclean, Sadie Ethel (1892–1989). Born in Glace Bay, Cape Breton, d/o Lauchlin, superintendent of the Sydney and Louisburg Railway, and Catherine (McKeagan) Maclean, she had ten months' CAMC experience when she joined the CAMCNS in Halifax in July 1918. She served in No. 11 CGH, No. 16 CGH and the CAMC Casualty Company. She was SOS in June 1919 and was living with her family in Glace Bay in 1921. She subsequently returned to Halifax and in 1934 married Dr. Thomas Henry MacDonald. They lived in Dedham and West Bedford, Massachusetts.

214. Macleod, Margaret Christine (1887–1919). Born in Dominion No. 6, Donkin, Cape Breton, d/o Duncan and Margaret (MacKeagan) Macleod, she was a 1911 graduate of the VGH School of Nursing and had a year's experience in the militia, serving in the CMH, when she joined the CAMCNS in Quebec City in September 1914. She went overseas with No. 2 CGH but fell ill in England and was sent home, but subsequently returned and served in No. 1 CGH, on HMHS *Letitia*, in No. 16 CGH, Granville Canadian Special Hospital, No. 13 CGH, No. 4 CGH and No. 1 CCCS when she fell ill again in February 1919. She was discharged for health reasons and returned home in June 1919. She was treated at CHH and then the Nova Scotia Sanatorium in Kentville, suffering from tuberculosis. She died there in December 1919. Oddly, she has two tombstones in St. Luke's cemetery: a private one and one provided by the Commonwealth War Graves Commission.

215. MacLeod, Marion (1893–1975). Born in Fox Brook, Pictou County, d/o George (deceased) and Ellen (Sinnis) MacLeod, Stellarton, Pictou County, she had a year's experience with the Harvard Surgical Unit at RAMC No. 22 General Hospital at Étaples when she transferred into the CAMCNS in London in June 1918. She served in No. 11 CGH and No. 14 CGH until returning to Halifax and being SOS in March 1919. She later moved to New York, where she married Blair Bonner, an automobile mechanic, until retiring to Middletown, Connecticut. Her brother, James MacLeod, declared in 1941 that she was "almost a stranger...as she had been away from home since her school days."[272] Her sister, Jessie Margaret MacLeod (1902–1941), was a nurse in the Second World War, serving at first with the Royal Canadian Medical Corps, then the RCAF station in Dartmouth until falling ill and dying from spinal meningitis in April 1941.

216. MacLeod, Sadie (1893–1946). Born in Baddeck, Victoria County, d/o Angus (deceased) and Mary (Gunn) MacLeod, she was a 1915 graduate of the VGH School of Nursing and was nursing in the CMH when she joined

the CAMCNS in October 1915. She served in No. 7 CSH, No. 4 CCS and the King's Canadian Red Cross Special Hospital at Bushy Park, London. She returned home in October 1918 and served in the Moxham Castle and Ross Convalescent Hospitals in Sydney until being SOS in May 1919. In November 1919 she married Dr. James Albert Currie, a Port Morien physician who had joined the CEF in May 1917 and but contracted rheumatic fever while at Camp Aldershot. He was treated at Moxham Castle Convalescent Hospital until being SOS in August 1918 as "physically unfit" and died of pulmonary tuberculosis in 1931. She then resumed nursing and served in CHH from 1942 to 1945.

217. MacLeod, Sadie Isabel (1889–1967). Born in New Haven, Victoria County, d/o Hector and Catherine (Hellen) MacLeod (both deceased), she was a graduate of the Winnipeg General Hospital School of Nursing and had three months' CAMC experience when she joined the CAMCNS in Halifax in June 1918, naming her brother John Joseph MacLeod as NOK. She went overseas in September 1918, served at the Shorncliffe CAMC Depot, No. 15 CGH and the CAMC Casualty Company. Then she was transferred home and SOS in April 1919. She nursed in Chicago for many years and was naturalized as an American citizen in 1930 but retired to live with a sister in Truro, Colchester County. Her brother Hector MacLeod enlisted in the 185th Battalion at the age of sixteen, claiming to have been born in 1898, and naming Sadie, who was then in England, as his NOK. He served in the 85th Battalion and was promoted to sergeant in December 1918.

218. MacNeil, Mary Eleanor (1882–1955). Born in Port Hood, Inverness County, d/o Daniel and Margaret Ellen "Maggie" (McDonald) MacNeil (deceased), she had sixteen months' CAMC experience when she joined the CAMCNS at Halifax in July 1918 and served in CHH and the Charlottetown Military Hospital until being SOS in May 1919. She moved to Boston and died there but is buried with her family in Halifax. Her father was a lawyer and Liberal MLA for Inverness (1886–1894) and a member of the Executive Council (1886–93). In November 1918 he was appointed a county court judge but died in an accident before taking office.

219. MacNeill, Mary Bell (1888–1976). Born in Ingonish, Victoria County, d/o Michael and Margaret (Cameron) MacNeill, Bridgeport, Cape Breton, she was a graduate of St. Joseph's Hospital School of Nursing. She was nursing in Montreal and had CAMC experience there when she joined the CAMCNS in December 1915. She served in No. 6 (Laval) CGH, the Moore Barracks Hospital at Shorncliffe, later designated to No. 11 CGH, No. 2 CSH and No. 14 CGH until being transferred in April 1919 to MD 6 and served at the Moxham Castle Convalescent Hospital in Sydney and the CHH. She was

SOS in September 1919 but remained in the CAMCNS and is thought to be the only Canadian First World War nurse who served also in the Second World War. She served as matron of CHH until 1945 and was awarded the Royal Red Cross 1st Class, the British War Medal, and the Victory Medal for her thirty years of service. She died at CHH in Halifax. Her brother, Angus MacNeill, a coal miner, enlisted in the 25th Battalion but was wounded in February 1916 and had arthritis and served as a stretcher bearer with No. 14 Field Ambulance. He was SOS in October 1919 and subsequently moved to Rosedale, Alberta.

220. Manning, Myra Ayer (1883–1971). Born in Wallace, Cumberland County, d/o William and Agnes (Betts) Manning (both deceased), she was nursing in Halifax and had two years' CAMC experience when she joined the CAMCNS in July 1918. She named her sister, Isabella, wife of James Craigie, a Nova Scotian who had moved to Haverhill, Massachusetts, as NOK. She served at CHH until being demobilized in October 1919, then moved to Brookline, Massachusetts, in 1926, was naturalized in 1943, and died there.

221. McCarthy, Mary Charlotte (1883–1968). Born in Colchester, England, d/o Thomas (deceased), a British army officer stationed in Halifax, and Eliza Anne (Dunn) McCarthy, she was a 1915 graduate of the VGH School of Nursing and had two years' CAMC experience when she joined the CAMCNS in December 1917. She served in No. 14 CGH and No. 9 CGH at Kinmel Park, then was transferred to Halifax, where she served in CHH and subsidiaries until being SOS in January 1920. She may have served as assistant supervisor in Sherbrooke Hospital, Sherbrooke, Quebec, before moving to New York City in 1923. She was joined by her mother after her father died in 1925. She retired in 1960 and settled in Dartmouth, Halifax County.

222. McCrea, Teresa Anna Carlotta (1888–1975). Born in Springtown, Ontario, d/o Joseph (deceased) and Caroline Teresa McCrea, she was nursing in Halifax and had thirteen months' CAMC experience when she joined the CAMCNS in August 1918. She served at CHH and CMH until being SOS in September 1919. She later moved to Pointe-Claire, Quebec.

223. McCurdy, Lillie Claire (1887–1980). Born in Old Barns, Colchester County, d/o James and Amelia (Archibald) McCurdy (both deceased). She listed her sister, Elizabeth McCurdy, as NOK and had CAMC experience when she joined the CAMCNS at Valcartier in September 1914. She served in No. 1 CGH and No. 2 CSH and was awarded the Royal Red Cross 2nd Class but resigned in November 1916 because of severe bronchitis. That same month she married Dr. Stuart Fisher, a physician from London, Ontario, who also served in No. 2 CSH, and they moved there.

224. McDonell, Mary "May" Elizabeth (1886–1937). Born in Enfield Station, Hants County, d/o Duncan and Esther (McCormick) McDonell, she was living in Halifax and had CAMC experience when she joined the CAMCNS in April 1917, naming her mother as NOK. She served in the MD 6 Training Depot and CHH and subsidiaries until being SOS in August 1919 as "medically unfit." In 1921 she was living at home and working on the family farm until 1926, when she married Thomas O'Donnell, a miner from Scotland, who had been a patient in the Nova Scotia Sanatorium in Kentville.

225. McIntosh, Margaret Isabelle (1875–?). Born in Halifax, Halifax County, d/o Robert and Ann (McLellan) McIntosh (both deceased), McLellan Mountain, Pictou County, she named her brother, Rev. John A. McIntosh, as NOK when she joined the CAMCNS in April 1915 in Montreal, where she likely studied nursing. She served in No. 1 CGH and No. 3 CGH, where she was mentioned in dispatches, No. 16 CGH, then the Canadian Forestry Corps Hospital at Lajoux. She returned to Halifax and was SOS in June 1919. In 1921, she appears to have nursed at Fraser's Point, a community southeast of Montreal, but subsequently moved to Vancouver, BC.

226. McKay, Alice Lettie (1881–1931). Born in Northfield, Lunenburg County, d/o Hibbert and Mary Abigail (Silver) McKay (both deceased), Blockhouse, Lunenburg County. In 1903 she had married Alex Foshay Fuller, a farmer from Hantsport, but they divorced before she joined the CAMCNS. She was a 1911 graduate of the VGH School of Nursing. She also studied nursing in Boston and had CAMC experience when she joined the CAMCNS in Halifax in February 1915. She served in No. 2 CGH and CGH No. 3. at Le Tréport, No. 2 CCCS at Shorncliffe and No. 12 CGH. She struggled with health issues, however, and was transferred to Halifax in May 1919 for further treatment in Pine Hill Convalescent Hospital, the CMH and CHH until being SOS as "medically unfit" in August 1919. In 1921 she married Joseph Zwicker, a farmer from New Germany, who enlisted in the 112th Battalion in February 1916 but served overseas in the 18th Canadian Machine Gun Company and the Canadian Cavalry Machine Gun Squadron.

227. McKinnon, Euphemia (1875–1970). Born in Whycocomagh, Inverness County, d/o Archibald and Isabella (MacRae) McKinnon, Sydney, Cape Breton County, she was a 1912 graduate of St. Joseph's School of Nursing and the Jeffery Hale Hospital—now the Jeffery Hale Minor Emergency Clinic—in Quebec City and shaved ten years off her date of birth when she joined the CAMCNS in October 1915. She served in No. 7 CSH, the Canadian Convalescent Hospital at Uxbridge, and No. 4 CGH until being transferred in April 1918 to MD 6, where she reverted to the CAMC and served in the Moxham Castle and Ross Convalescent Hospitals in Sydney

until being SOS in March 1919. She continued nursing in Sydney in 1923 but was nursing at the Harbor Veterans Hospital in Brooklyn, New York, in 1927. Then she was appointed the first registered nurse to serve in the North Victoria Cottage (Buchanan Memorial) Hospital in 1943.

228. McLennan, Katharine (1892–1975). Born in Sydney, Cape Breton, d/o John and Louise (Bradley) (deceased) McLennan, stepdaughter of Grace Seely (Henop) McLennan, and sister-in-law of Dr. Henry Kendall, she had studied art in Paris before the war and in 1916 joined the Société Française de Secours aux Blessés Militaires, the French Red Cross Society, in 1916. She also served in the Hôpital de l'Alliance in Yvetot; the No. 109 Hôpital Auxiliaire in Pont-Audemer; a hospital referred to as Hôpital d'Évacuation 18 at Vasseny; the Hôpital Militaire at Pontoise; the Hôpital Militaire, Caserne de Cavalière, and a German hospital at Bad Schwalbach, a spa town twenty kilometres from Wiesbaden. During that time, she made sketches of the soldiers in the hospitals, took many photographs and wrote letters home describing her experiences, including complaining of the lack of trained nurses. After the war she supported the Red Cross and the VON in Cape Breton but focused on promoting the history of the eighteenth-century French fortress at Louisbourg until the federal government agreed in the 1960s to restore it. She was invested in the Order of Canada and received an honorary degree from St. Francis Xavier University. Her father was a Montreal-born industrialist who had moved to Sydney, Cape Breton, and was a senior executive with the Dominion Iron and Steel Company that also owned the region's coal mines, then acquired the *Sydney Daily Post* (now the *Cape Breton Post*) newspaper and during the war was president of the Cape Breton Patriotic Fund, served on the Military Hospitals Commission, and was appointed to the Senate in 1916. Her brother, Hugh McLennan, joined the 5th Battery, 2nd Brigade, Canadian Field Artillery in August 1914 and was killed at Ypres in April 1915.

229. McLeod, Annie Tremaine (1887–1976). Born in Sydney, Cape Breton, d/o Dr. William and Hattie (Tremaine) McLeod and a granddaughter of Rev. Hugh McLeod, a prominent minister who served as the third Moderator of the Presbyterian Church in Canada, she was nursing at the Rockhead Infectious Diseases Hospital in Halifax and had three months' CAMC experience when she joined the CAMCNS in April 1916. She served in No. 9 CSH, the Moore Barracks Hospital at Shorncliffe (later designated No. 11 CGH), No. 3 CSH, No. 2 CGH and No. 12 CGH. She returned to Halifax and was SOS in June 1919 and subsequently married George Stanway, a banker from Charlottetown, PEI, who had served as a captain in the 105th Battalion, which went overseas, merged with the 104th Battalion, then

was absorbed by the 13th Reserve Battalion. He and Annie moved in the 1920s to Burnaby, British Columbia. Her father had studied medicine in New York and represented Cape Breton in the House of Commons from 1879 to 1882, was appointed medical superintendent of quarantine in Sydney, president of the Cape Breton Medical Society, and organized and commanded the Sydney Battery of Field Artillery.

230. McLeod, Isabel Gordon (1887–1988). Born in New Lairg, Pictou County, d/o Alexander and Margaret (Gordon) McLeod, Lansdowne Station, she had CAMC experience when she joined the CAMCNS in Montreal in August 1916. She served in the Westcliffe Canadian Eye and Ear Hospital, the CAMC Depot, No. 2 CGH, No. 14 CGH and No. 9 CGH and was transferred to MD 6. She was SOS in August 1919, moved to Vancouver, and married David Hazlewood, a nurse, who had served as an orderly in No. 7 CGH and No. 12 CGH.

231. McManus, Laura Mabel (1885–1951). Born in Memramcook, New Brunswick, d/o Jeremiah and Sarah (Pettipas) McManus (both deceased), and sister of Lila Teresa McManus, she was nursing in Halifax. She had a year's CAMC experience and named her brother, Dr. Charles Burriss McManus, as her NOK when she joined the CAMCNS in July 1918. She served in the CMH until being SOS in February 1919 and married Dr. John A. MacDonald in Halifax. They later moved to Montreal, Quebec.

232. McManus, Lila Teresa (1889–1955). Born in Memramcook, New Brunswick, d/o Jeremiah and Sarah (Pettipas) McManus (both deceased), and sister of Laura Mabel McManus, she was nursing in Halifax. She had eighteen months' CAMC experience and named her brother, Dr. Charles Burriss McManus, as her NOK when she joined the CAMCNS in July 1918. She served in CHH until being SOS in July 1919. In November 1920 she married Edgar Mingo, who had joined the 17th Battalion as a lieutenant in September 1914 but served as a captain in the 13th Battalion, was twice wounded and repatriated to Halifax for convalescent treatment at CHH and Pine Hill Convalescent Hospital. He subsequently became a broker in Halifax.

233. McNeill, Margaret Blanch (1890–1968). Born in Aylesford, Kings County, d/o Aaron and Annie (Gates) McNeill, she joined the QAIMNS in England and served for a year in Malta, then returned to London in May 1918 and transferred into the CAMCNS. She served in No. 10 CGH until returning home and was SOS in August 1919. In 1925 she married Stanley Bellamy in Islington, then a suburb of Toronto, Ontario, but they later lived in Jacksonville, Florida, and Perquimans County, North Carolina, until divorcing in 1938, after which she moved to Astor, Lake County, Florida.

234. Mills, Alice Muriel (1888–1945). Born in Truro, Colchester County, d/o Alfred Creighton and Alice Caroline (Grant) Mills, she was a 1912 graduate of the VGH School of Nursing and joined the CAMCNS in February 1915. She served in No. 2 CGH at Le Tréport and No. 16 CGH until being granted leave in Canada, then resigned in May 1918. She was one of the thirty-two Nova Scotian nurses who went to Boston that year to help with the influenza epidemic.
235. Mills, Ethel Rosamond (1887–1965). Born in Halifax, d/o William and Alice (Jones) Mills, she was nursing there and had twenty-six months' CAMC experience when she joined the CAMCNS in August 1918. She served in CHH until being SOS in June 1919. Three months later she married Brewer Robinson in Boston. He was from Summerside, Prince Edward Island, and had served overseas with No. 2 Heavy Battery, Canadian Field Artillery, then was a fox rancher, mayor of Summerside (1936–37) and a member of the PEI legislature (1939–45) while serving overseas with Canadian Legion War Services and was a senator from 1945 until his death in 1949.
236. Mitchell, Jean Marguerite (1892–1988). Born in Bridgeport (Dominion), Cape Breton County, d/o Henry and Janet (MacDougall) Mitchell, she joined the CAMCNS in October 1915 and served in No. 7 CSH. She resigned in April 1918 to marry Lieutenant Colonel John Scott, an Australian who commanded the 21st Australian Infantry Battalion, in London. They moved to Sydney, Australia, and she remained there after their divorce in 1926.
237. Moreshead, Eleanor Gorrill (1891–1985). Born on Prince Edward Island, d/o (William) Daniel and Mary (Gorrill) Moreshead, Sydney River, Cape Breton, she was a graduate of the RVH School of Nursing and had CAMC experience in Montreal when she joined the CAMCNS in November 1916. She served in No. 9 CSH, No. 12 CGH, No. 7 CGH, No. 15 CSH, the CAMC Casualty Company at Shorncliffe and No. 16 CGH, then returned home and was SOS in June 1919. She resumed nursing in Montreal and in 1922 married Dr. Gerald Carlton Melhado, a surgeon from Bermuda who had studied medicine at McGill University. He joined No. 4 CGH with the rank of captain in May 1916 and served overseas at Salonika until contracting influenza and was transferred to Ste. Anne's Military Hospital at Saint-Anne-de-Bellevue in Montreal in April 1919. They lived in Saint-Jacques, Quebec.
238. Morrison, Anna May (1887–1998). Born in Gabarus, Cape Breton, d/o Roderick, a merchant and ship owner, and Melinda (Matheson) Morrison, she was a 1912 graduate of the VGH School of Nursing and was nursing in Halifax and had CAMC experience when she joined the CAMCNS in May 1918. She served in the MD 6 Training Depot and CHH until being SOS in

July 1919. Two months later she married Dr. Daniel Finlayson MacInnis of Middle River, Victoria County, a 1918 graduate of the Dalhousie Medical School who had been senior houseman at the VGH in 1917 at the time of the Halifax explosion, then joined the CAMC and served in CHH. She retired after they settled in Shubenacadie, Hants County.

239. Morrison, Daisy Dean (1882–1965). Born in Springfield, Annapolis County, d/o John and Roseann (Mason) Morrison, she was a 1916 graduate of the VGH School of Nursing. She joined the CAMC and nursed in the CMH for two years, then joined the CAMCNS in February 1918, at which point she rather oddly added thirteen years to her date of birth. She served in No. 14 CGH, No. 9 CGH and No. 15 CGH until returning home and being SOS in July 1919. She briefly nursed in Vancouver before returning to Halifax and serving in the VGH, where she met and married Henry Percy Davies, of Montreal, who had enlisted in the Royal Highlanders in October 1916 but fell ill in Halifax before going overseas and was discharged in January 1918. They moved to Montreal, where she continued nursing, but later lived in Brockville, Ontario. Their son, John Frederick Davies, joined the RCAF in 1941, rose to the rank of colonel and commanded several military bases over the years.

240. Morrison, (Mary) Ethel (1877–1954). Born in Pictou, Pictou County, d/o Malcolm and Lydia (Rood) Morrison, she moved with her family to Victoria, British Columbia, in the late 1890s. She was a graduate of the Vancouver General Hospital's School of Nursing and had CAMC experience when she joined the CAMCNS in Victoria in September 1915. She served in No. 5 CGH at Salonika and No. 1 CGH in France and England, was awarded the Royal Red Cross 2nd Class and was twice mentioned in dispatches. She remained in England after the war, nursing in Canadian medical units in Shorncliffe and Liverpool until returning and serving briefly in Ottawa and at the Esquimalt Military Hospital until April 1920. After taking courses in public health nursing, she was a school nurse in Esquimalt, retiring in 1945. In 1938 she published a brief article of her wartime experience in *The Canadian Nurse* and kept a photo album that became the subject of a book entitled *Battlefront Nurses in WW I* (2009) written by her niece, Maureen Duffus.[273]

241. Morrison, Myrtilla Grey (1888[274]–1933). Born in Londonderry, Colchester County, d/o Samuel and Jane (Holmes) Morrison, she had CAMC experience when she joined the CAMCNS in September 1916. She served in England at the Westcliffe Canadian Eye and Ear Hospital, Nos. 1, 2, 5, 9 and 15 CGHs and the King's Canadian Red Cross Special Hospital. She returned to Halifax in June 1919 and was SOS but continued nursing until her retirement.

242. Mosher, Eva Maude (1885–1964). Born in Moosehead, Halifax County, d/o George and Sarah (Atkins) (deceased) Mosher, Halifax, she was a 1908 graduate of the VGH School of Nursing and had served as a head nurse in the Beth Israel Hospital in Roxbury, Boston. She appears to have served with American Red Cross nurses to organize public health work in France with the RAMC No. 1 CSH at Rouen.[275] In 1915 she transferred into the CAMCNS and served in No. 1 CGH at Étaples, the CAMC Depot at Shorncliffe, the Canadian Red Cross Hospital at Buxton, and No. 4 CGH until being transferred to MD 6 because of health issues and was SOS in April 1919. She moved to British Columbia and in 1922 married James Wilfred Watt, an engineer. They lived in Nelson, BC; Seattle, Washington; Port Alberni, BC; and finally Vancouver in 1952. Her brother, Newman Hall Mosher, served briefly with the MD 6 Engineering Depot in Halifax.

243. Mosher, Lyda Theresa (1889–1932). Born in Bridgeport, Connecticut, d/o Robert (deceased) and Mary (Mahoney) Mosher and stepdaughter of Monson Kilcup. The family moved to Kentville in the 1890s, but she studied nursing in New York City. She was working as a VON nurse in Truro and, according to the Kentville *Advertiser*, would be "greatly missed in the VON work in Colchester and especially in connection with her school inspection"[276] when she joined the CAMCNS in Halifax in July 1916. She initially named her mother as NOK but later changed that to her sister, Lois Mosher, because her mother was in poor health (and died in May 1917). She served in the DCRC, No. 1 CGH, the CAMC Training Depot at Shorncliffe, No. 16 CGH and No. 10 CGH but had recurrent health issues, including neurasthenia. She also served twice on hospital ships, the *Northland* in February 1917 and the *Letitia* in April 1917, including during a leave in Canada to June 1917. Upon her return to England, she was ill with gastroenteritis in the Canadian Red Cross Special Hospital at Buxton in October/November 1917 and the Kitchener Military Hospital in November 1918. She resigned in January 1919 and was invalided home for treatment at Ste. Anne's Military Hospital in Saint-Anne-de-Bellevue, Montreal. She then returned to Halifax before moving to Peabody and Holyoke, both in Massachusetts, but died in Leavenworth, Kansas, in 1932.

244. Mulcahy, Grace Mary (1887–1974). Born in Halifax, Halifax County, d/o Patrick and Catherine "Addie" (Winsor) (deceased) Mulcahy, she had twenty-six months' CAMC experience when she joined the CAMCNS in August 1918. She served at the CMH and CHH until being SOS in November 1919. She moved to Vancouver, where in 1925 she married Edward Rathje, an American-born farmer from Lacombe, Alberta, who had been conscripted in May 1918 and served in the Alberta Regiment Depot Battalion

in England. Her brother, Arthur Mulcahy, who was living in Worcester, Massachusetts, enlisted in the 236th Battalion in Fredericton in June 1917 but served overseas in the 13th Battalion, then moved to Boston.

245. Murray, Ann Elizabeth (1881–1959). Born in Durham, Pictou County, d/o Donald and Jane (Campbell) Murray (both deceased), she was a graduate of the Worcester State Hospital School of Nursing in Worcester, Massachusetts. She had nineteen months' experience in the Harvard Surgical Unit with the RAMC No. 22 General Hospital at Étaples when she transferred into the CAMCNS in London in July 1918, naming her sister, Charlotte, as her NOK. She served in the Canadian Convalescent Officers' Hospital at Matlock Bath, No. 9 CGH at Kinmel Park and No. 11 CGH, then returned to Halifax in July 1919 and was SOS in August 1919. In 1920 she married Samuel Byrod Fortenbaugh, a lawyer, and they lived in Schenectady, New York, for several years, then retired in Palo Alto, California.

246. Murray, Emma Blanche (1883–1978). Born in Truro, Colchester County, d/o James and Emmeline (Archibald) Murray, she had CAMC experience when she joined the CAMCNS in Halifax in April 1917. She served in the Kitchener Military Hospital (redesignated No. 10 CGH in September 1917), No. 9 CGH and the Canadian Convalescent Hospital at Bear Wood until returning to Halifax and being SOS in May 1919. She moved to Vancouver and married Thomas McRae in 1921, but they moved to Blaine and Seattle, in Washington, then Los Angeles and La Crescenta-Montrose, California.

247. Mury, Simon (1891[277]–1960). Born in West Arichat, Richmond County, s/o Laurent and Admila (Boudrot) Mury, he declared that he was a nurse and may have graduated from either the VGH School of Nursing or St. Joseph's Hospital's School of Nursing at Glace Bay when he joined No. 7 CSH in November 1915. He was approved by Lieutenant Colonel John Stewart but only as a private. He served with No. 7 at Le Havre until October 1916, until being transferred to No. 1 CGH at Étaples and promoted to corporal in July 1918. He was SOS in April 1919 and moved to Alberta, where he farmed, then was a schoolteacher and later lived at Lafond.

248. O'Brien, Marcella Agnes (1871–1953). Born in Antigonish, Antigonish County, d/o James and Alice (Grant) O'Brien (both deceased), she named her brother, John Sarsfield O'Brien, the Conservative member of the House of Assembly for Antigonish from 1913 to 1916, as NOK when she joined the CAMCNS in April 1916, despite being forty-five years old. She served in No. 9 CSH and No. 16 CGH, then returned to Halifax and was SOS in July 1919. She married Hector MacNeil, a steel plant manager in Sydney Mines and a widower. They were living in Los Angeles in 1940 but later lived in Woodside (Dartmouth), Halifax County.

249. O'Callaghan, Mary (1877–1922). Born in Halifax, Halifax County, d/o James and Annie (Graham) O'Callaghan (both deceased), Sydney, Cape Breton County, she was living in Sydney with her sister, Maggie O'Callaghan, whom she named her NOK, and had fifteen months' CAMC experience when she joined the CAMCNS in November 1918, despite being forty-one years of age. She served in the Moxham Castle and Ross Convalescent Hospitals in Sydney until being SOS in January 1919. She died in Sydney three years later.

250. O'Leary, Catherine[278] Mary (1894–1966). Born in Pugwash, Cumberland County, d/o Thomas (deceased) and Charlotte "Lottie" (Cox) O'Leary, she had six months' CAMC experience when she joined the CAMCNS in August 1918. She served at CHH until being SOS in June 1919, then moved to New York City and in November 1920 married Charles Tuttle of Wallace Bay, Cumberland County. He had joined the 40th Battalion as a lieutenant in October 1915 but served as a captain in the 60th Battalion, was wounded and transferred to Halifax for convalescent treatment. They lived in Yonkers, New York, and Cincinnati and Rocky River, Ohio, but later returned to Halifax.

251. Paget, Gertrude White (1891–1941). Born in Hazel Hill, Guysborough County, d/o Frederick (deceased) and Eliza (White) Paget, she had CAMC experience when she joined the CAMCNS in Montreal in May 1917. She served in England in the Canadian Officers' Convalescent Hospital at Broadstairs, No. 4 CGH, No. 3 CGH, the Granville Canadian Special Hospital at Buxton, the Canadian Convalescent Officers' Hospital at Matlock Bath, No. 11 CGH and No. 16 CGH, then returned to Halifax and was SOS in August 1919. Her mother and siblings had moved to San Francisco in January 1918, and Gertrude joined them there but later moved to Siskiyou County in northern California. Her brother, Frederick Paget, a student, served overseas in the 11th Canadian Engineers Battalion and rose to lieutenant in 1918.

252. Paton, Florence Mary[279] (1885–1968). Born in Westville, Pictou County, d/o David and Evaline (Spinney) Paton and sister of Mary Steele Paton, she had CAMC experience when she joined the CAMCNS in Halifax in June 1917, naming her father as NOK. She served in the Westcliffe Canadian Eye and Ear Hospital, RAMC No. 3 CSH, the CAMC Casualty Company at Shorncliffe and No. 15 CGH, then returned to Halifax and was SOS in April 1919. She later moved to Waltham, Massachusetts, and lived with her other sister, Julia, and her family, who had moved there, and her sister Mary Steele Paton. Their brother, Arthur Paton, enlisted in the 25th Battalion and was wounded on the Somme in September 1916.

253. Paton, Mary Steele (1883–1922). Born in Westville, Pictou County, d/o David and Evaline (Spinney) Paton and sister of Florence Mary Paton, she joined the CAMCNS in Montreal in April 1916, naming her father as NOK. She served in the Granville Canadian Special Hospital, No. 2 CGH, No. 6 CGH, No. 4 CGH and No. 12 CGH, then returned home and was SOS in July 1919. She later moved to Waltham, Massachusetts, and lived with her sisters Florence and Julia Paton, who had all moved there.

254. Perry, Dorothy Bronte (1882–1965). Born in Barton, Digby County, d/o Anthony "Augustus" and Orlinda (Haines) Perry, she studied nursing in Newton, Massachusetts, then was living in Montreal and had CAMC experience when she shaved three years from her date of birth and joined the CAMCNS in June 1917. She served in No. 4 CGH, No. 12 CGH, No. 9 CGH and No. 11 CGH, then returned to Halifax and was SOS in August 1919. She subsequently lived with her brother, Augustus, sister Hattie, and mother in Barton and continued nursing until 1940.

255. Perry, Helen Hastings (1887–1967). Born in Yarmouth, Yarmouth County,[280] d/o Albert (deceased) and Mary (Booth) Perry, she studied nursing in Newton, Massachusetts, and nursed in the American Red Cross Military Hospital in London for five months until transferring into the CAMCNS in March 1918, naming her brother, Albert Booth Perry, as NOK. She served in No. 16 CGH and the CAMC Casualty Company at Shorncliffe but had health problems and was invalided home in March 1919. After obtaining further treatment at Ste. Anne's Military Hospital in Montreal, she moved to New York in 1920 and continued nursing until she married George Conley in 1931. They lived in Harrietstown, New York, and Lake Clear, New York.

256. Piercey, Annie Olive (1884–1959). Born in Dutch Village, Halifax County, d/o Charles and Eleanor (Drysdale) Piercey, she was a 1915 graduate of the VGH School of Nursing and nursed at the Rockhead Infectious Diseases Hospital in Halifax until May 1917 when she joined the CAMCNS, naming her brother, Charles Piercey, as NOK. She served in the DCRC and Red Cross hospitals in France until resigning and returning home in July 1918. She nursed in the VGH for a time, then in Dr. Anthony Mader's private maternity hospital in Halifax and continued nursing until 1934 when she retired to Middle Musquodoboit. Her brother was a businessman in Sydney, Cape Breton, and had ten years' experience in the Canadian Field Artillery when he joined the CEF at Valcartier with the rank of captain, was awarded the DSO, and rose to the rank of lieutenant colonel commanding the 1st Brigade but fell ill and died on November 18, 1918.

257. Porter, Mary Agnes "Nellie" (1869–1964). Born in Wilmot, Annapolis County, d/o Rev. William Henry and Elizabeth (Marshall) (deceased) Porter, Toronto,

Ontario, and wife of Dr. Alexander Carmichael Robertson, she shaved twenty-two years off her date of birth and joined the CAMCNS in May 1917, naming her brother, George Dana Porter, as NOK. She served in the MD 2 base hospital until falling ill and was SOS in September 1918. Her husband also joined the CAMC in July 1917, and was posted to Edmonton, where he died in 1919. Her brother, also a physician, joined the CAMC with the rank of captain in August 1915 and served in Toronto. She subsequently moved to White Rock, British Columbia.[281]

258. Prest, Violet Ella (1894–1975). Born in Mooseland, Halifax County, d/o William and Henrietta (Glencross) Prest, she was a 1917 graduate of the Waterbury Hospital School of Nursing in Waterbury, Connecticut, and had two months' CAMC experience in Halifax when she joined the CAMCNS in July 1918. She served in the CMH and CHH in Halifax and was SOS in October 1919. She was living with her parents in 1921 but in 1924 was in Boston, where she married John Lovitt Golden, a Nova Scotian who had served briefly in the 1st Depot Battalion in Halifax in May 1918. They moved to Quincy, Massachusetts, and later Portland, Maine.

259. Purcell, Marie Louise (1887–?). Born in Halifax, Halifax County, d/o William and Catherine (Low) Purcell, Purcell's Cove, she lived in Quebec City before the war but was living with her parents in Halifax and had CAMC experience when she joined the CAMCNS in June 1918, listing her mother as NOK. She served in No. 11 CGH but developed serious health problems and was invalided home in May 1919 for further treatment at Ste. Anne's Hospital in Montreal. She married Joseph William Spencer, who was born in Ireland but had grown up in the Coombe Orphanage at Hespeler, Ontario. He served in the 111th and 4th Battalions until falling ill and was SOS as "medically unfit" in October 1918. They lived in Montreal and had a son, Joseph William Spencer, who was baptised in 1930, by which time Joseph appears to have moved to Toronto, where he died in 1970.[282] She returned to Halifax and in 1949 was nursing at the Children's Hospital but in 1958 was living in Canton, Ohio.

260. Rathbone, Annie Simpson (1879[283]–1953). Born in Grand Pré, Kings County, d/o Ida and Annie Rathbone, Lockhartville, she moved to Winnipeg in 1896 and became the first district nurse with the Margaret Scott Nursing Mission, then was one of the original organizers of the Anti-Tuberculosis Society and was appointed matron of the Ninette Sanatorium for three years. She subsequently moved to the United States for a nursing position and served overseas with the American Red Cross. Invalided back to Canada at the end of the war, she nursed at Gibsons, British Columbia, until retiring to Winnipeg in 1949 and dying there.[284]

261. Redmond, Charles Alfred (1878–1925). Born in Sheet Harbour, Halifax County, s/o Peter (deceased) and Ellen (Purcell) Redmond and husband of Margaret "Minnie" (Hechler) Redmond, he was a 1905 graduate of the VGH School of Nursing but described himself as a labourer when he married in 1914. He had three years' CAMC experience when he enlisted in No. 7 CSH in November 1915 with the rank of sergeant, naming his wife as NOK. He served as an orderly, not a nurse. He returned to Halifax in April 1919 and served in CHH until being SOS in January 1920, then was working as a labourer in East Chezzetcook, Halifax County, in 1921. His brother, Joseph Earl Redmond, was conscripted in June 1917 and served with the Canadian Railway Troops in England and France.
262. Renshaw, Lilian Cameron. *See* Dunbar, Lilian Cameron.
263. Rice, Frances Augusta (1884–1962). Born in Weymouth, Digby County, d/o Thomas and Clara (Payson) Rice, Yarmouth, she was a 1912 graduate of the VGH School of Nursing and was nursing in the CMH in Halifax when she joined the CAMCNS in December 1915. She served overseas in No. 7 CSH, the Granville Canadian Eye and Ear Hospital, the Shorncliffe Military Hospital and No. 2 British Stationary Hospital. She returned to Halifax in May 1918, served in CHH and CMH, and was awarded the Royal Red Cross 2nd Class. She was SOS in April 1920 and continued nursing until retiring in 1952.
264. Richardson, Edith Louisa (1880–1949). Born in Belfast, Ireland, d/o Clement and Louisa (Mansell) Richardson, who had emigrated in 1911 with their children to a farming community near Winnipeg, she studied nursing in the United States, possibly at Saint Vincent Hospital or the University of Massachusetts, both of which are in Worcester, a place that she visited in 1924. She was nursing in Halifax and had four months' CAMC experience when she joined the CAMCNS in May 1917, naming her sister, Ruth, wife of Henry Greenley, as NOK, perhaps because her parents were elderly and were living with Ruth and her family. Edith served in No. 16 CGH, No. 8 CSH and No. 2 CGH, then returned to Halifax and served at CHH and subsidiaries until being SOS in January 1920. She continued nursing until retiring in 1943 and died in Canning, Kings County.
265. Rose, Lenora "Nora" Elizabeth (1884–1964). Born in Dartmouth, Halifax County, d/o Henry and Maria (Merson) Rose (both deceased), she had CAMC experience and shaved three years off her date of birth when she joined the CAMCNS in Toronto in February 1916, naming her uncle, Thomas Merson, as NOK. She served in No. 16 CGH, No. 2 CGH, No. 1 CGH, No. 2 CCCS and the CAMC Casualty Company, returning home in September 1919. She then moved to Kingston, Ontario, presumably to marry Dr. John Edward

Kain, a physician who had joined the CEF and served in the Shorncliffe CAMC Depot, No. 1 CGH, No. 2 CCCS, the Canadian Forestry Corps Detention Hospital at Alençon, the CAMC Casualty Company and No. 16 CGH. They married in 1923 and subsequently moved to Hartford, Connecticut.

266. Ross, Elizabeth Belle (1878–1953). Born in Demerara, Guyana, d/o Rev. Francis and Elizabeth (MacGillivray) Ross, New Glasgow, Pictou County, she joined the Société Française de Secours aux Blessés Militaires, the French Red Cross Society, in Belgium and served as matron of nurses in the American Ambulance Hospital at Neuilly, Paris, before transferring into the CAMCNS in London in February 1916. She served as acting matron in the DCRC and was promoted to matron of No. 10 CGH in January 1918. She was brought to the notice of the Secretary of War and was awarded the Royal Red Cross 1st Class, the British War Medal and the Victory Medal. She returned home in October 1919 and subsequently nursed at the Woman's Hospital in New York City and in Philadelphia until retiring to Ottawa. Her father had spent twenty-two years in pastorates in the West Indies and served as a chaplain in the South African War.

267. Ross, Catherine "Kathryn" Dorothy (1895–1967) Born in Bridgeville, Pictou County, d/o Cyrus and Christy (Grant) Ross and niece of Thomas Cantley, president of the Nova Scotia Steel and Coal Company, member of parliament from 1925 to 1930, and senator from 1935 to 1945. Her family had moved to Winnipeg, and she was a 1917 graduate of the Winnipeg General Hospital School of Nursing. She had CAMC experience when she joined the CAMCNS in March 1918 and served in No. 10 Manitoba Military Hospital until being SOS in August 1919. She subsequently went to China to help open a hospital and serve as superintendent of the Chengtu School of Nursing sponsored by the American Methodist Church.[285] She also taught nursing at the Rockefeller Hospital in Beijing. In the Second World War, she served as matron of the CMH and the Sydney Military Hospital, then was transferred to Winnipeg's Fort Osborne Barracks Hospital. She later served with the United Nations Relief and Rehabilitation Administration in Europe and was in charge of a new hospital in Lahore, Pakistan.[286] She then moved to Halifax and nursed there until retiring in June 1966. Her brother, William Field Ross, served in the 10th Battalion and was wounded in March 1918.

268. Ross, Vivian Russell (1884–1958). Born in North Sydney, Cape Breton, d/o Rev. Jeptha Gilead (deceased) and Margaret (Salter) Ross, she was nursing in Halifax and had eight months' CAMC experience when she joined the CAMCNS in July 1918, naming her sister, Katherine Isabel Ross, as NOK. She served in CHH until being SOS in March 1919, then resumed nursing in North Sydney until retiring in 1940.

269. Schaffner, Marion Parker (1895–1978). Born in Middleton, Annapolis County, d/o Leonard and Ann (deceased) (Elliott) Schaffner, and sister of Muriel Campbell Schaffner (*See* #271), she was nursing in Halifax and had fifteen months' CAMC experience when she joined the CAMCNS in July 1918, naming her father as NOK. She served at CHH and subsidiaries until being SOS in August 1919, then moved to Boston. In 1920 she married Joseph Tagen, a businessman who had served briefly in the US Army in 1918, and they lived in Braintree, Massachusetts. After his death in 1946, she moved to Avon, Connecticut.

270. Shaffner, Mary "Minnie" Victoria (1890–1965). Born in South Farmington, Annapolis County, d/o Charles and Jessie (deceased) (Phinney) Shaffner and stepdaughter of Isabella (Harris) Shaffner, Middleton, Annapolis County, she was a 1912 graduate of Acadia University and may have trained as a nurse in the United States. She is thought to have served in Halifax during the war and may have returned to the United States until the 1950s when she was resident superintendent of the Nova Scotia Sanatorium in Kentville and was living in Digby, Digby County. She retired in Wolfville, Kings County. Her brother, Louis Shaffner, served overseas in the 29th Battalion and was killed at Loos in August 1917.

271. Schaffner, Muriel Campbell (1896–1966). Born in Middleton, Annapolis County, d/o Leonard and Ann (deceased) (Elliott) Schaffner, and sister of Marion Parker Schaffner (*See* #269), she was nursing in Halifax and had two months' CAMC experience when she joined the CAMCNS in August 1918, naming her father as NOK. She served in the CMH and CHH until being SOS in May 1919. In August 1919 she married Vernon Beckwith Durling of Lawrencetown, Annapolis County, who had served overseas in the 73rd and 42nd Battalions. They lived in Middleton until 1928, when their son, George, died, after which they moved to Boston and divorced in Florida the same year. She subsequently lived in Natick, Massachusetts, and was naturalized in 1945.

272. Sedgewick, Jessie Ann Middleton (1890–1958). Born in Middle Musquodoboit, Halifax County, d/o William (deceased) and Anne (Leedham) Sedgewick, she was nursing in Montreal when she joined the CAMCNS in April 1915, naming her brother, George Sedgewick, a Toronto lawyer, as NOK. She served in No. 3 CGH, the Shorncliffe CAMC Depot, No. 16 CGH and the Granville Canadian Special Hospital, then was posted to Canada in February 1919 and served in Ste. Anne's Military Hospital in Montreal until July 1919. In 1920 she married Charles Lightfoot Roman, whose grandfather had fled from enslavement in Maryland to Canada via the Underground Railroad. Charles had obtained a science degree at Fisk University in Nashville and

was studying medicine at McGill University when he joined No. 3 CGH in February 1915 at a time when Black Canadians were not generally welcomed in the CEF, serving as an orderly with the rank of private and later sergeant. When the government called on all medical and dentistry students serving overseas to return home to complete their studies, he returned to McGill in June 1917 and graduated in 1919. Jessie and her husband lived in Valleyfield, Quebec, where she was working alongside him when he became one of the first industrial doctors in the province, employed by Montreal Cottons Limited, a division of the Dominion Textile Company, and became a leader in the field of occupational medicine.

273. Shannahan, Mary Catherine (1892–1951). Born in Halifax, Halifax County, d/o William and Catherine (Walsh) Shannahan (both deceased), she was a 1915 graduate of the VGH School of Nursing and had twenty-three months' CAMC experience when she shaved four years from her date of birth and joined the CAMCNS in December 1917, naming her aunt, Margaret Walsh, as NOK. She served in England in the Granville Canadian Special Hospital at Buxton, No. 3 CGH, the Shorncliffe CAMC Casualty Company, No. 16 CGH and No. 15 CGH and contracted influenza twice, then was transferred to Halifax and served in CHH from August 1919 until January 2020, when she was SOS. She continued nursing in the United States and Halifax until retiring in 1946.

274. Shaw, Annie Cornelia. *See* Strong, Annie Cornelia.

275. Skerry, Agnes Elizabeth (1886–1969). Born in Waverley, Halifax County, d/o William and Ellen (Knox) Skerry, she was a 1912 graduate of the VGH School of Nursing and took postgraduate courses in pediatrics at Boston Floating Hospital.[287] She joined the American Red Cross and served overseas in the war, then married Archibald Whicher of Ohio, and they lived in San Francisco, California.

276. Skerry, Annie Adelaide Blanch (1884–1957). Born in Waverley, Halifax County, d/o Thomas and Sarah (Hessian/Hanshan) Skerry, she had CAMC experience when she joined the CAMCNS in February 1917 and served in No. 8 CSH at Westenhanger, No. 12 CGH at Hastings, and No. 13 CGH, then was transferred to MD 6 in February 1919 and was SOS in July 1919. In 1922 she married Joseph Horne, a farmer from Enfield, on the border of Hants and Halifax Counties, but they later moved to Waverley, Halifax County, where he worked at the Halifax shipyards. He died in April 1957, and she followed a month later.

277. Smiley, Jessie Beatrice "Trix" (1885–1968). Born in Salmon River, Halifax County, d/o Matthew and Mary (Turner) Smiley, Port Dufferin, Halifax County, she was a 1915 graduate of the VGH School of Nursing, had six

months' CAMC experience, and was serving at CHH when the Halifax Explosion took place. She joined the CAMCNS in April 1918 and served briefly at the Westcliffe Canadian Eye and Ear Hospital at Shorncliffe, where she met Dr. Rodger Nicholls, a doctor from Edmonton. They married in January 1919 and resigned in July 1919, moving to Edmonton, where he resumed his practice and she worked as his office nurse.

278. Smith, Catherine Sarah (1890–1977). Born in Piedmont, Pictou County, d/o Hugh and Mary Ann (Cumming) Smith, Sydney, Cape Breton County, she was a 1914 graduate of the VGH School of Nursing and was nursing at the Brookland Street Hospital in Sydney, when she went to Halifax and joined the CAMCNS in November 1915. She served in No. 7 CSH, No. 1 CGH, No. 3 CGH, No. 15 CGH and the DCRC. She returned home in March 1919 and served at CHH and the CMH until being SOS in March 1920. She moved to Vancouver, BC, and in 1924 was appointed superintendent of Mayo Landing Hospital, Yukon. There she married John Dempster, the commanding officer of the Mayo RCMP Detachment. The Dempster Highway from Dawson City to Fort McPherson is named after him.

279. Smith, Mabel Elizabeth "Eliza" (1873–1957). Born in Economy, Colchester County, d/o Richard (deceased) and Josephine (Thompson) Smith, Parrsboro, Cumberland County, she was scheduled to go to England in May 1915 but actually went in December 1916, perhaps because her mother had moved to Ottawa and died in September 1916. She served in No. 1 CGH until suffering anaemia and bronchitis and was given leave to Canada until February 1917, then served in No. 11 CSH, No. 1 CGH, the Canadian Red Cross Special Hospital at Buxton, the Granville Canadian Special Hospital, the Canadian Officers' Hospital at Broadstairs, No. 4 CGH, No. 8 CSH and No. 7 CGH, until being SOS in July 1919. She later lived in Kelowna, BC, but was buried in a cemetery in Parrsboro. Her brother, Don Cecil Smith, enlisted in the 219th Battalion but served in the 85th Battalion and was killed at Passchendaele in October 1917 and is honoured on the Menin Gate Memorial at Ypres.

280. Stevens, Annie Jane (1890–1962). Born in Wallace Grant, Cumberland County, d/o Arad and Catherine (MacLennan) Stevens and sister of Louise Myrtle Stevens (*See* #281), Bayhead, Colchester County, she likely was a graduate of the Montreal General Hospital's School of Nursing because she was nursing in Montreal when she joined the CAMCNS in July 1918. She served in the Drummond Military Convalescent Hospital in Montreal, the Shorncliffe CAMC Depot, No. 10 CGH and No. 4 CGH, then returned to Canada and was SOS in July 1919. In 1926 she married Roy James McNutt, a farmer, and they lived in Wallace Grant, and later Richmond, Cumberland County.

281. Stevens, Louise Myrtle (1888–1985). Born in Wallace Grant, Cumberland County, d/o Arad and Catherine (MacLennan) Stevens and sister of Annie Jane Stevens (*See* #280), she likely was a graduate of the McGill University School of Nursing because she was nursing in Montreal when she joined the CAMCNS in April 1915. She served in No. 3 (McGill) CGH, No. 1 CGH, No. 4 CCCS, No. 10 CSH and No. 4 CGH, then returned home and was SOS in July 1919. She resumed nursing in Montreal until her retirement but was buried in Tatamagouche, Colchester County.
282. Stewart, Margaret Wood (1891–1980). Born in Digby, Digby County, d/o Walter (deceased) and Louisa (Raymond) Stewart, she was nursing in Halifax and had eight months' CAMC experience when she joined the CAMCNS in July 1918, naming her brother, James Alvin Stewart, as NOK. She served in No. 12 CGH and No. 15 CGH and was SOS at Halifax in July 1919. She was nursing in Sydney in 1921 when she married Dr. Donald Angus MacLeod, a 1911 graduate of the Dalhousie Medical School, who served in No. 7 CSH in October 1915 and was wounded at Passchendaele in October 1917. He continued his practice in Glace Bay and later Sydney, and she was a homemaker and a mother of two children. At some point after his death in 1938, she moved to Halifax and was nursing at the Children's Hospital in 1949. They are buried together in Sydney.
283. Strong, Annie Cornelia (1887–1970). Born in Canning, Kings County, d/o Everard and Elizabeth (Rand) Strong, she had three years and three months' CAMC experience in Halifax and Quebec when she joined the CAMCNS at Valcartier in September 1914. She served as matron of No. 1 CGH, in No. 2 CGH, No. 2 Clearing Station, No. 13 CGH and No. 2 CSH, was twice mentioned in dispatches and was awarded the Royal Red Cross 1st Class. In October 1915 she married Greville Havergal Shaw, an Englishman who had emigrated to Canada and was an officer in the Royal Canadian Engineers. He served at Halifax and in Quebec before the war, then in the 12th Battalion and was promoted to major, then very briefly acting lieutenant colonel until being killed at Valenciennes in November 1918. Annie served as matron of the Quebec Military Hospital in 1919 and retired in Ottawa. Her brother, Harold Edward Strong, was conscripted in February 1918 and served in No. 17 Reserve Battalion in England but was discharged as "medically unfit" in April 1918. Her husband's brother, Giles Havergal Shaw, served as a lieutenant in the British 5th (Territorial) Battalion and was killed in action in April 1917.
284. Sullivan, Mary Margaret (1890–1966). Born in Halifax, Halifax County, d/o Maurice and Elizabeth (Dunlay) Sullivan, she was nursing in Halifax and had three months' CAMC experience when she joined the CAMCNS

in July 1918. She served at CHH and subsidiaries until being SOS in May 1919. She continued nursing in Halifax and married Charles Patterson, a machinist, in November 1921. They lived in Dartmouth. He had joined the army in September 1916 and served overseas in the 3rd Battalion, Canadian Railway Troops, until falling ill in December 1918 and was invalided to Halifax in May 1919. He died in 1931.

285. Sutherland, Roberta (1877–1959). Born in Halifax, Halifax County, d/o James and Isabel (Norrie) Sutherland (both deceased), she was nursing in Halifax and had two years and five months' CAMC experience when she shaved six years off her date of birth and joined the CAMCNS in August 1918, naming her sister, Christina Maud Sutherland, as NOK. She served in CHH, the CMH, the Camp Aldershot hospital and the Pine Hill Convalescent Hospital until being SOS in May 1919. Her death certificate states that she retired from nursing in 1918, but she was still nursing in Halifax in 1923.[288]

286. Tait, Mary (1876–1963). Born in Hercall (High Ercall), Shropshire, England, d/o William and Hannah Tait, Wellington, Shropshire, she was nursing in Halifax and had CAMC experience when she joined the CAMCNS in May 1917. She served in No. 10 CSH, No. 14 CGH, the Granville Canadian Special Hospital, the Shorncliffe CAMC Casualty Company and No. 16 CGH. She was SOS in Halifax in August 1919 and may be the Mary Tait who lived and died in Salmon Arm, British Columbia.

287. Thomas, Lalia Elizabeth (1885–1943). Born in Canard, Kings County, d/o William and Susannah (Borden) Thomas (both deceased), she was a 1915 graduate of the VGH School of Nursing when she joined the CAMCNS in October 1915, naming her sister, Ella, wife of Edmund Daley, a Baptist minister in Halifax, as her NOK. She served in No. 7 CSH and RAMC No. 2 Stationary Hospital but developed health issues and was transferred to MD 6 in May 1919. She nursed at CHH and subsidiaries until being discharged in January 1920. She continued nursing at CHH and later was superintendent of the Halifax Infants Home until retiring in 1927.

288. Thompson, Edith Alexandria (1869–1959).[289] Born in Halifax, Halifax County, d/o William (deceased) and Martha (Elliott) Murray, and wife of Rev. William Thompson, she studied nursing at the VGH and was nursing in Halifax when she shaved nine years from her date of birth and joined the CAMCNS in April 1916, naming her sister, E. M. Murray, as NOK. She served in No. 9 CSH, the Granville Canadian Special Hospital, No. 2 CGH, the Canadian Convalescent Hospital at Bear Wood, the Westcliffe Canadian Eye and Ear Hospital, and No. 13 CGH. She was SOS in March 1919 and resumed nursing in Halifax until moving to Jacksonville, Florida, where she died and is buried.[290]

289. Thompson, Ethel Elaine (1882–1959). Born in Nine Mile River, Hants County, d/o Charles and Isabella (Walker) Thompson, she was nursing in Halifax and had a year's CAMC experience when she joined the CAMCNS in April 1918. She served overseas in No. 4 CGH and No. 12 CGH and was awarded the Royal Red Cross 2nd Class. She was SOS in August 1919 and returned to Halifax, then moved to Calgary in 1921 and settled finally in Jacksonville, Florida.

290. Thompson, Wilhelmina "Irene" (1889–1975). Born in Glencoe, Pictou County, d/o James and Melinda "Linda" (McMillan) Thompson, she studied maternity at the Wesson Maternity Hospital in Springhill, Massachusetts, and was also a 1915 graduate of the VGH School of Nursing. She joined the CAMCNS in December 1915 and served in No. 7 CSH, the Shorncliffe Canadian Eye and Ear Military Hospital, No. 4 Casualty Clearing Station, then was transferred to Halifax in May 1919. She served in CHH and subsidiaries until being SOS in December 1919 and continued nursing at CHH and the Nova Scotia Sanatorium until 1923, when she married Stanley Williams Spicer, a dentist in Canning. They later moved to Kentville, Kings County, and retired to Advocate Harbour, Cumberland County. Her brother, William Percy Thompson, served in the 5th Battalion and was killed at Vimy Ridge in April 1917. Their son, Stanley Thompson Spicer, served in the merchant marine and the Canadian army in the Second World War, published eleven books and several magazine articles on the age of sail in the Maritimes, and received an honorary degree from Acadia University in 2000.

291. Tout, Dora Oliva (1882–1948). Born in Halifax, Halifax County, d/o William and Selina (Atkinson) Tout (both deceased), she had five months' CAMC experience when she joined the CAMCNS in April 1918, naming her sister, Florence Taylor, as NOK. She served in No. 11 CGH, No. 14 CGH and No. 16 CGH, returning home and being SOS in September 1919. She continued nursing in Halifax in 1923, Liverpool in 1935 and Truro in 1940, retiring to Halifax in 1945.

292. Trivett, Jean Dorothy (1891–1986). Born at sea, d/o Rev. Samuel and Catherine (Jennings) Trivett, when they were returning from England to Lower Stewiacke, Colchester County, where her father was an Anglican priest. Before settling in Nova Scotia, in 1878 they had emigrated to Alberta, where her father established a mission and residential school on the Blood Reserve and wrote a Blackfoot dictionary. He then served parishes in Manitoba, Michigan, and Nova Scotia.[291] Jean had eight months' CAMC experience when she joined the CAMCNS in August 1918 in Halifax and served in CHH and subsidiaries. She was SOS in February 1919 and in 1921 was nursing in Toronto. In subsequent years she nursed in Quebec and Ontario, retiring in Brantford, Ontario.

293. Tupper, Adruenna "Addie" Allen (1860–1916). Born in Yarmouth, Yarmouth County, d/o George (deceased) and Mary (Raymond) Allen, stepdaughter of Rufus Trefry (deceased), and widow of Stanley Tupper. She attended the Acadia University Seminary (collegiate course) and was a graduate of the Concord Hospital School of Nursing in Connecticut. She moved with the family to Bridgewater in the 1890s and nursed there. When she joined the CAMCNS at Quebec City in September 1914, she shaved ten years from her date of birth and went overseas with the first contingent. She served in No. 2 CGH until August 1915, when her health began to fail and she was given leave in November 1915 to return home on a hospital ship. While in Bridgewater, she gave talks about her experiences and raised money for Canadian convalescent soldiers in hospitals in England. When she returned to England in December, she served at the Granville Canadian Special Hospital at Ramsgate for four months. She then returned to France in February 1916 and was awarded the Royal Red Cross 1st Class. She returned to England in November 1916 and served in the Hillingdon House Convalescent Hospital at Uxbridge but fell ill with pneumonia and died in December 1916.

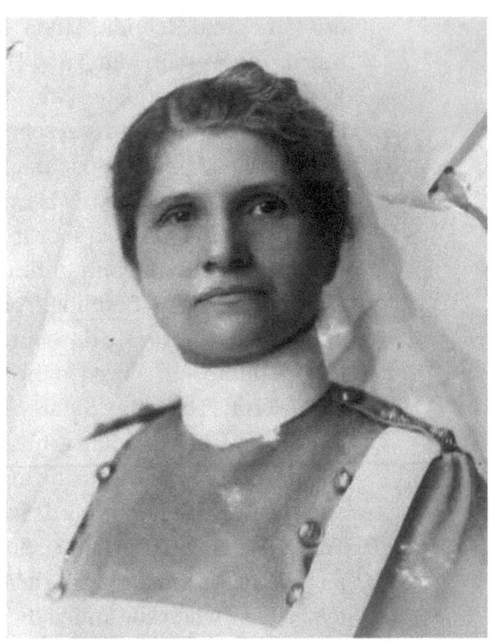

Adruenna Tupper.
[COMMONWEALTH WAR GRAVES COMMISSION]

294. Urquhart, Abbie Ross (1890–1956). Born on a British ship in New York Harbour, d/o Frederick (deceased) and Leila (Cummings) Urquhart, Truro, Colchester County, and stepdaughter of Alfred Davidson, she was living in Halifax and had five months' CAMC experience when she joined the CAMCNS in August 1918, naming her mother, who was living in New Rochelle, New York, as NOK. She served in the CMH in Halifax until being SOS in December 1918, then moved to New Rochelle. Her brother, Charles William Urquhart, served overseas in the 29th (Vancouver) Battalion and was killed at the Somme in September 1916.

295. Urquhart, Charlotte "Lottie" (1888–1987). Born in New Glasgow, Pictou County, d/o John and Catherine (Robertson) Urquhart, she was a 1909 graduate of the Boston State Hospital School of Nursing and the Montreal General Hospital School of Nursing in 1913. She had CAMC experience when she joined the CAMCNS in January 1916. She served with No. 6 CGH at Troyes but was transferred to No. 1 CGH at Étaples and was there when it was bombed on the evening of May 18, 1918. One officer, one nurse and forty-five other ranks were wounded, eight patients were killed, and thirty-one others were wounded. Matron Edith Campbell reported Urquhart's "gallantry and devotion to duty...when four bombs fell on her wards. Regardless of danger, she attended to the wounded. Her courage and devotion were an inspiring example to all." The result was that Campbell, Urquhart, and four other nurses were awarded the Military Medal for "bravery on the field."[292] She also served in No. 2 CGH and No. 7 CGH, both at Le Tréport, until returning to England and serving briefly in No. 4 CGH and No. 15 CGH. After being demobilized in Halifax in July 1919, she returned to Montreal but later moved to Vancouver where three of her sisters lived. She worked for an insurance broker for several years until marrying Reginald Seys, who had served overseas in the 14th Brigade, Canadian Field Artillery. Her brother, Edwin Urquhart, enlisted in the 17th Battalion in September 1914 but served in the 13th Battalion and was wounded in October 1915.

296. Urquhart, Susan Hope (1891–1962). Born in Tatamagouche, Colchester County, d/o Andrew (deceased) and Annie (McKenzie) Urquhart, she joined the CAMCNS at Halifax in May 1918. She served in the MD 6 Training Depot, the CMH and CHH until being SOS in July 1919. She subsequently nursed in New York but later moved to Montreal and lived with her sister, Margaret, widow of Duncan MacLennan, who had died in 1932.

297. Van Buskirk, Katharine "Kitty" (1894–1984). Born in Dartmouth, Halifax County, d/o George and Agnes (Elliott) Van Buskirk, she attended a convent school, then went to Boston in 1913 to study nursing at the Massachusetts General Hospital School of Nursing. While there, she became a close friend of Helen Dore Boylston, who went on to become a well-known novelist and used their experiences in many of her books. One of her main characters was Kit Van Dyke, modelled on Katherine. In 1915 Van Buskirk and Boylston joined the Harvard Surgical Unit and served at the RAMC No. 22 General Hospital at Étaples, an experience that Boylston described in *"Sister": The War Diary of a Nurse* (New York, 1927). After the war Van Buskirk nursed in New York until 1920 when she and Boylston joined the American Red Cross and were assigned to a hospital in Tirana, Albania,

but didn't stay long because of the unstable and dangerous environment, which Boylston described in an article in the *Atlantic Monthly* in November 1925. They were then assigned to Krakow, Poland, but the situation there was no better, and they returned to New York in February 1921, where Van Buskirk worked as a psychiatric nurse. She subsequently was assistant superintendent of the Faulkner Hospital in Boston. In 1935 she returned home and married Karl Woodbury, a Halifax dental surgeon, and died in Middleton, Annapolis County. Her brother, Lawrence Elliott Van Buskirk, joined the 5th Divisional Signal Company with the rank of lieutenant in 1916 but suffered neurasthenia and was SOS in April 1918.

298. Viets, Carolyn Winnifred (1888–1962). Born in Digby, Digby County, d/o Rev. John (deceased), a descendant of Connecticut Loyalists, and Jane (Roberts) Viets, she studied nursing in the United States, then went to England and joined the TFNS. She nursed at the Beech House Military Hospital in London and the DCRC until transferring into No. 2 CSH in February. She was awarded the Royal Red Cross 2nd Class in March 1916. She was then promoted to matron-in-chief for duty overseas and was posted to No. 4 CGH at Salonika in November 1916. She fell ill in January 1917 and returned to England in September 1917, then served briefly in No. 16 CGH, the Canadian Red Cross Officers Hospital in London, the Canadian Forestry Corps Hospital at Beech Hill (London) and the Canadian Red Cross Special Hospital at Buxton, then back to Beech Hill until returning to Halifax in April 1919 where she served briefly at CHH. After being SOS in May 1919, she moved to Lincoln, Massachusetts, in 1921. Three years later she married Henry Corbitt, a fruit farmer from Annapolis Royal who had enlisted in the 214th Battalion in 1916 but served overseas in the 5th Battalion. They farmed in Penticton, British Columbia, and she died in Kaleden, Okanagan-Similkameen Regional District. Her brother Alexander Griswold Viets enlisted in the Princess Patricia's Canadian Light Infantry in December 1914 and was blinded in action at Ypres in May 1915. Another brother, Robert Botsford Viets, a lawyer who was the private secretary of the minister of finance in Ottawa, joined the 207th Battalion but served in the 38th Battalion and was wounded in December 1917.

299. Wall, James Joseph (1884[293]–1971). Born in Goshen, Guysborough, s/o James (deceased) and Margaret (McPherson) Wall who had moved to Antigonish, he was a 1907 graduate of the VGH School of Nursing and joined No. 9 CSH in Antigonish in March 1916, not as a nurse but as a private soldier (service #534442), serving as an orderly with the rank of staff sergeant. He developed health issues in 1918 and was SOS in July 1919. In 1923 he

married Mary Theresa Lynch (*See* #159), and they lived in Antigonish, where he was a butcher.

300. Walsh, Marguerita "Rita" Mary (1894–1964). Born in Halifax, Halifax County, d/o William and Bridget (Walsh) Walsh, she had CAMC experience when she joined the CAMCNS in April 1917. She served in No. 16 CGH, the Granville Canadian Special Hospital, No. 6 (Laval) CGH in France and No. 15 CGH until returning to Halifax in July 1919. She reverted to the CAMC and served in CHH until being SOS in November 1919. She continued nursing in Halifax until 1962. Her brother, John Walsh, was a commercial traveller in Winnipeg when he was conscripted in October 1917 and served the 8th Battalion in England and France.

301. Walters, Emma Jane (1894–1976). Born in Granton, Pictou County, d/o Edward (deceased) and Catherine (McQuaig) Walters, Westville, Pictou County, she was a graduate of St. Joseph's Hospital School of Nursing and joined the CAMCNS in October 1915. She served in No. 7 CSH and No. 1 CGH until returning in May 1919 to Halifax, where she served at CHH until being SOS in January 1920. She continued nursing until 1925, when she moved to Boston and then to New York City, where she married Lorne Bayliss, a Nova Scotian from New Glasgow, Pictou County, in 1927. He had been conscripted in April 1918 and briefly served in the Nova Scotia Regiment's 1st Depot Battalion until being released because he was an American citizen. They later retired in Kissimmee, Florida.

302. Watson, Agnes Maud (1883–?). Born in Falmouth, Jamaica, d/o John and Jane (Smith) Watson (both deceased), she and her two sisters—Maude (Beatrice) and Mabel (*See* #303)—followed their brother, David Watson, who had moved to Halifax in 1898 to study medicine at Dalhousie University. He married Emma Morton, and they lived in Bedford, Halifax County, until 1905 when they returned to Jamaica, but returned in 1914 and he died in February 1918. She was a 1910 graduate of the VGH School of Nursing and was nursing in Halifax with sixteen months' CAMC experience at the CMH when she joined the CAMCNS in May 1917, naming her sister Maude as her NOK, and served in the Shorncliffe Military Hospital, No. 9 CGH, and No. 3 CGH until resigning in May 1918. Maude served at the RVH in Montreal and the CAMCNS in Toronto from September 1918 to October 1919 and later moved to Niagara Falls and died there.[294]

303. Watson, Mabel Margaret (1884–1955). Born in Falmouth, Jamaica, d/o John and Jane (Smith) Watson (both deceased), and sister of Agnes (*See* #302), Maude, and David Watson. She was a 1909 graduate of the VGH School of Nursing and had CAMC experience in the CMH when she joined the CAMCNS in December 1916, initially listing another sister, Dora Watson of

Tobermory, Scotland, as her NOK but later changing that to yet another sister, Estelle (Watson) Carver, who lived in New York and later Plainfield, New Jersey. Mabel served in the Shorncliffe Military Hospital, No. 8 CGH, No. 3 CGH, No. 1 CGH, the Shorncliffe CCCC, and No. 11 CGH but developed serious health issues and returned to Halifax in June 1919. She was treated at the CMH but was diagnosed with tuberculosis and was treated at the Nova Scotia Sanatorium in Kentville. She later lived in New York City and Hanover, New Hampshire, where she taught nursing at the Mary Hitchcock Memorial Hospital, adjacent to Dartmouth College.

304. Whidden, Mary Douglas (1888–1964). Born in Masstown, Colchester County, d/o James and Jane "Jennie" (Faulkner) Whidden, Truro. She shaved two years from her date of birth and had CAMC experience when she joined the CAMCNS at Halifax in December 1917. She served with the MD 6 Training Depot and CHH until being SOS in July 1919, then returned to Truro and served as a school nurse.

305. White, Katherine Elizabeth (1890–?). Born in Moser River, Guysborough County, d/o Elizabeth J. White, Bishop's Falls, Newfoundland, she had four months' experience in the QAIMNS in England when she transferred into the CAMCNS in August 1917. She served briefly in the DCRC, then was posted to No. 10 CSH, returning to Halifax in June 1919 and was SOS in July 1919. She subsequently lived and nursed in Alert Bay, British Columbia.

306. Williams, Maysie Ellen (1889–1930). Born in Musquodoboit Harbour, Halifax County, d/o Lawrence and Mary (Madore) (deceased) Williams, she was a 1911 graduate of the VGH School of Nursing and was nursing with the VON in Toronto when she joined the CAMCNS in Halifax in October 1915. She served in No. 7 CSH, No. 2 CGH, RAMC No. 2 Stationary Hospital—which was taken over by No. 2 CSH in September 1915—and No. 3 CGH but fell ill with tonsilitis and was transferred to Halifax in May 1919 and had surgery. She served in CHH until being SOS in February 1920. She subsequently moved to Prince Rupert, British Columbia, where she married Thomas Allen, who was born in Iowa, in 1921. They moved to Smithers, BC, then Edson, Alberta.

307. Wishart, Joyce Thomson (1888–1924). Born in Saint John, New Brunswick, d/o Allison and Alice (Thomson) Wishart (deceased), she may have studied nursing in Saint John but was living with her parents and was nursing in Halifax, where her father was a physician, when she joined the CAMCNS in February 1915. She served in No. 1 CSH and No. 1 CGH in France until falling ill in May 1917. She was treated in a number of hospitals in England until being posted to the Canadian Red Cross Special Hospital in Buxton. There she met Archibald Maclean, a lawyer from Saskatoon, who had

joined the 11th Battalion at Valcartier in August 1914. Upon arrival in England in October 1914, it was designated a reserve battalion and absorbed other battalions until January 1917, when he was promoted to the rank of major and second in command of the Canadian Discharge Depot at Buxton, where they met. Joyce and Archibald were SOS in May 1918, married in June 1918, and returned home and lived first in Battleford and then in Lloydminster, Saskatchewan, until his death in 1921. She returned to Saint John and, remarkably, died three years later.

308. Young, Anna Teresa (1885–1961). Born in Dartmouth, Halifax County, d/o Joseph and Clara (Halls) Young, she was a 1916 graduate of the VGH School of Nursing and was nursing in Yarmouth when she joined the CAMCNS in April 1916, naming her brother, Rev. W. E. Young, as NOK. She served in No. 9 CSH, the DCRC, No. 12 CGH, No. 7 CGH, No. 8 CGH, No. 11 CGH and the Granville Canadian Special Hospital at Buxton. She returned to Halifax and was SOS in August 1919 and served in CHH. Then she was a private duty nurse in New York City until returning to Yarmouth by 1923 and later moving to Dartmouth, Halifax County.[295]

309. Young, Frances Rand (1889–1970). Born in Kentville, Kings County, d/o William (deceased) and Margaret (Rand) Young, Kentville, she was a granddaughter of Leander Rand, a local businessman, who served in the House of Assembly from 1886 to 1890 and married Olivia Ann Borden, making Frances related to Sir Robert Borden, Sir Frederick Borden, Allison Borden and Katherine MacLatchy (*See* #206), the matron of No. 3 (McGill) CGH and principal matron for MD 6. Frances was a 1916 graduate of the RVH School of Nursing in Montreal and served at the Royal Canadian Navy Hospital in Halifax. When it was damaged in the Halifax Explosion, she served on the USS *Old Colony*—a former passenger ship that the US Navy was sending to England but was in drydock awaiting boiler repairs and became a temporary hospital ship—and anonymously published an account of her experience. In December 1919 she married Bellenden Hutchison, a physician born in Mount Carmel, Illinois, who had joined the CEF in 1915 and served overseas as medical officer with the rank of captain in the 75th Battalion. He was awarded both the Military Cross and the Victoria Cross for his bravery on the battlefield and for treating German casualties as well as Canadians. After the war they lived in Cairo, Illinois, but his Victoria Cross is displayed in the Toronto Scottish Regiment's museum in Mississauga, Ontario.

310. Young, Josephine Matilda (1880–1929). Born in West Petpeswick, Halifax County, d/o William "Henry" and Emily Ann (Baker) Young and sister of Rose Olga Young (*See* #311), she was a 1906 graduate of the VGH School of

Nursing and had two years and seven months' CAMC experience with the CMH when she shaved four years from her date of birth and joined the CAMCNS in December 1915. She served in Halifax at the CMH, CHH and the MD 6 Training Depot until being SOS in September 1919. In October 1919 she moved to Detroit, Michigan, to marry Francis John Splatt, an accountant from Brantford, Ontario, who had moved there. Remarkably, he is confused with William Francis Splatt, who was also living in Brantford and had joined the 13th Battalion Royal Highlanders at Valcartier in September 1914 and was killed in action in April 1915.[296] Both Josephine and Francis died very young: she in Detroit in 1929, and he in a car accident in 1930. She is buried there, but he is buried in Chatham, Ontario.

311. Young, Rose Olga (1886–1934). Born in West Petpeswick, Halifax County, d/o William "Henry" and Emily Ann (Baker) Young and sister of Josephine Matilda Young (***See*** #310), she was a 1909 graduate of the VGH School of Nursing and had nursed in Detroit, Michigan, and Calgary, Alberta, before returning home. She was night supervisor at the VGH, then nursed at the CMH when she joined the CAMCNS in October 1915. She served in No. 7 CSH and No. 14 CGH until returning to Halifax in May 1919 and served at CHH until being SOS in January 1920. She subsequently moved to Detroit, where she married Percy S. Smith. She died in 1934 of tuberculosis in the Queen Alexandra Sanatorium in London, Ontario, and was buried in Detroit.

Appendix A

Nova Scotia Matrons

1.	Margaret Macdonald (*See* #181)	Matron-in-Chief
2.	Louise Brock (*See* #27)	No. 2 CSH and No. 4 CGH
3.	Elizabeth Doyle (*See* #73)	CMH
4.	Margaret "Pearl" Fraser (*See* #98)	*Llandovery Castle* Hospital Ship (acting matron)
5.	Harriet Graham (*See* #110)	Canadian Officers' Red Cross Hospital, London
6.	Laura Hubley (*See* #135)	No. 7 CSH
7.	Jessie Jaggard (*See* #139)	No. 3 CSH, Lemnos
8.	Janet Macdonald (*See* #176)	No. 2 CGH
9.	Sarah MacIsaac (*See* #194)	No. 9 CSH
10.	Katherine MacLatchy (*See* #206)	No. 3 CGH
11.	Elizabeth Ross (*See* #266)	No. 10 CGH
12.	Annie Strong (*See* #283)	Quebec Military Hospital, Quebec City
13.	Carolyn Viets (*See* #298)	No. 1 CSH

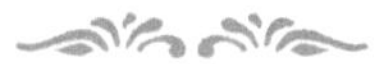

Appendix B

Canadian Nurses Who Died In Service
(Nova Scotians are in italics)

1915	*Jessie Jaggard*, No. 3 CSH
	Mary Frances Munro, No. 3 CSH
1916	*Neil MacLean*, 25th Battalion
	Addie Tupper, No. 2 CGH
1917	Sarah Garbutt, No. 16 CGH
	Etta Sparks, No. 7 CGH
1918	Jean Alport, No. 4 CGH
	Miriam Baker, No. 15 CGH
	Dorothy Baldwin, No. 3 CSH
	Christina Campbell, No. 5 CGH, *Llandovery Castle*
	Ainslie Dagg, No. 15 CGH
	Lena Davis, No. 4 CGH
	Carola Douglas, *Llandovery Castle*
	Alexina Dussault, *Llandovery Castle*
	Minnie Follette, *Llandovery Castle*
	Agnes Forneri, No. 8 CGH
	Margaret Fortescue, *Llandovery Castle*
	Margaret Fraser, Matron, *Llandovery Castle*
	Minnie Gallaher, *Llandovery Castle*
	Matilda Green, No. 7 CGH
	Victoria Hennan, No. 9 CGH
	Myrtle Hunt, Halifax Infirmary
	Jessie Jarvis, Cogswell Military Hospital
	Lenna Mae Jenner, Shorncliffe

	Ida Kealy, No. 1 CGH Margaret Lowe, No. 1 CGH
	Katherine Maud Macdonald, No. 1 CGH
	Rebecca MacEachen, CAMC
	Jessie McDiarmid, No. 5 CGH, *Llandovery Castle*
	Evelyn McKay, No. 3 CGH
	Mary McKenzie, *Llandovery Castle*
	Rena McLean, No. 2 CSH, *Llandovery Castle*
	Agnes Macpherson, No. 3 CSH
	Henrietta Mellett, No. 15 CGH
	Eden Pringle, No. 3 CSH
	Nellie Grace Rogers, Davisville Military Hospital (Toronto)
	Ada Ross, No. 1 CGH
	Mae Belle Sampson, *Llandovery Castle*
	Gladys Irene Sare, *Llandovery Castle*
	Anna Stamers, *Llandovery Castle*
	Jean Templeman, *Llandovery Castle*
	Alice Trusdale, CAMC
	Dorothy Pearson, VAD, served in hospital near London
	Gladys Wake, No. 1 CGH
	Anna Whitley, No. 10 CSH
1919	Margaret Baker, CAMC
	Ernestine Champagne, No. 8 CGH
	Petty Gertrude Donaldson, No. 1 CGH
	Grace Grant, CAMC
	Jessie King, No. 1 CGH
	Agnes McDougal, No. 10 CSH
	Rebecca McIntosh, No. 9 CGH
	Margaret MacLeod, No. 2 CGH
1920	Mary McGinnis, CAMC
1921	Isobel Cumming, No. 1 CGH
1922	Bessie Hanna, No. 3 CSH
	Caroline Green, CAMC HS

Endnotes

Preface

1. Cynthia Toman, *Sister Soldiers of the Great War: The Nurses of the Canadian Army Medical Corps* (UBC Press, 2016), 12.
2. Veterans Affairs Canada, "The Nursing Sisters of Canada." veterans.gc.ca/en/remembrance/those-who-served/women-veterans/nursing-sisters.
3. J. G. Adami, *War Story of the Canadian Army Medical Corps* (Musson Book, 1918), 235; Toman, *Sister Soldiers*, 39.
4. Toman, *Sister Soldiers*, 39.
5. Ibid.
6. Ibid., 40. Toman identifies six trained Newfoundland nurses who joined the QAIMNS—Bertha Forsey, Frances Maitland Frew, Grace Gardner, Isabel Holden, Maysie Parsons, and Katherine White—but she failed to include Elsie Doyle and incorrectly included Grace Gardner, Frances Cron and Martha Loder, making the number four.
7. Ibid. *See* Terry Bishop Stirling, "'Such Sights One Will Never Forget': Newfoundland Women and Overseas Nursing in the First World War," in Sarah Glassford and Amy J. Shaw, eds, *A Sisterhood of Suffering and Service: Women and Girls of Canada and Newfoundland During the First World War* (UBC Press, 2012), 130. The Newfoundland & Labrador in the First World War website says, rather unhelpfully, only that there were "about 175 women who served overseas as graduate nurses or with the Voluntary Aid Detachment." heritage.nf.ca/first-world-war/articles/nl-in-the-first-world-war.php.
8. Toman, *Sister Soldiers*, 68–72.
9. John Williams, *The Other Battleground: The Home Fronts: Britain, France and Germany, 1914–18* (Chicago, 1972), 253.

10. They were Louise Hopkins, Madeleine Jaffray, Mabel Joice, Annie Matthews, Margaret McIntyre, Helen McMurragh, Florence Morris and Laura Robinson. All were trained nurses. *See* Marlena Wyman, "Bluebird: Madeleine Jaffray." theprairieline.wordpress.com/2018/12/06/bluebird-madeleine-jaffray/.
11. *See* Linda Quiney, "'Filling the Gaps': Canadian Voluntary Nurses, the 1917 Halifax Explosion, and the Influenza Epidemic of 1918," *Canadian Bulletin of Medical History* 19:2 (2002), 351–74. doi.org/10.3138/cbmh.19.2.351. For the experience of one VAD, Bessie Hall of Bridgewater, see her wartime diary in Margaret Conrad, Toni Laidlaw and Donna Smith, eds, *No Place Like Home: Diaries and Letters of Nova Scotia Women 1771–1938* (Formac Publishing, 1988), 251–60. She had completed her BA at Dalhousie University in 1915 but gave up a teaching position in October 1918 to serve in CHH, hoping to get an overseas posting. She didn't and went on to earn a PhD at Bryn Mawr College in Pennsylvania in 1929 and was a social worker in the United States.
12. Susan Mann, "Where Have All the Bluebirds Gone? On the Trail of Canada's Military Nurses, 1914–1918," *Atlantis* 26:1 (Fall/Winter 2001), 37. atlantisjournal.ca/index.php/atlantis/article/view/1498. According to Mélanie Morin-Pelletier, "more than seventy nurse veterans found positions in the growing field of public health." "'At Peace with the Germans, but at War with the Germs': Canadian Nurse Veterans after the First World War," in Tim Cook and J. L. Granatstein, eds, *Canada 1919: A Nation Shaped by War* (UBC Press, 2020), 199.
13. *See* Brian Tennyson and Roger Sarty, *Guardian of the Gulf: Sydney, Cape Breton, and the Atlantic Wars* (University of Toronto Press, 2002).
14. *See* Alice Kelly, "'Can One Grow Used to Death?' Deathbed Scenes in Great War Nurses' Narratives," in Kellen Kurschinski, Steve Marti, et al, *The Great War: From Memory to History* (WLU Press, 2015), 329–49.

Introduction

15. David Rayside, "Rayside, Edith Catherine," *Dictionary of Canadian Biography,* vol. 17, University of Toronto/Université Laval, 2003–. biographi.ca/en/bio/rayside_edith_catherine_17E.html.
16. Bill Rawling, *Death Their Enemy: Canadian Medical Practitioners and War* (AGMV Marquis, 2001), 55–6.
17. Alexandra Minna Stern, "The Public Health Service in the Panama Canal: A Forgotten Chapter of US Public Health," *Public Health Chronicles*, 120:6 (November–December 2005), 675–79. doi.org/10.1177/003335490512000616.

18. Cynthia Toman, "Georgina Fane Pope." *The Canadian Encyclopedia*. Historica Canada. Article published December 13, 2007; Last Edited March 07, 2016. thecanadianencyclopedia.ca/en/article/georgina-fane-pope.
19. She died in 1938.
20. Guy Carleton Jones was born in Halifax, studied medicine at Dalhousie University, served in the South African War and was appointed director general medical services of the CAMC in 1906. He served overseas as assistant director of medical services, then was promoted to director in February 1915, based in London. He was the son of Alfred Gilpin Jones, a prominent businessman, member of parliament, and lieutenant governor of Nova Scotia in 1900–06.
21. Hannah Bentley, "Queen Alexandra's Imperial Military Nursing Service: A Study of Female Active Service During the First World War" (Unpublished PhD Thesis, University of East Anglia, 2021), 83, 87. ueaeprints.uea.ac.uk/id/eprint/85348. ***See also*** Rosemary Shields and Linda Shields, "Dame Maud McCarthy (1859–1949), Matron-in-Chief, British Expeditionary Forces France and Flanders, First World War," *Journal of Medical Biography* 24:4 (November 2016), 507–14. doi.org/10.1177/0967772013480610.
22 Veterans Affairs Canada, *Canada's Nursing Sisters* (Charlottetown, 2005), 6. veterans.gc.ca/en/remembrance/those-who-served/women-veterans/nursing-sisters.
23. Susan Mann, *The War Diary of Clare Gass, 1915–1918* (McGill-Queen's University Press, 2000), xix.
24. Gillian Woodford, "McGill's WWI Doctors and Nurses: A Proud but Bitter Legacy," *McGill Health E-News*, November 29, 2017. healthenews.mcgill.ca/mcgills-wwi-doctors-and-nurses-a-proud-but-bitter-legacy/.
25. Mann, *War Diary*, xxi; Woodford, "McGill's WWI Doctors and Nurses."
26. In 1921 the Nova Scotia Hospital affiliated with the VGH and the Grace Maternity Hospital to provide the third year, during which students were assigned to the VGH for six months and the Grace Maternity Hospital for three months. *Nursing Education in Nova Scotia* (1921). forms.msvu.ca/library/tutorial/nhdp/schools/NSH.htm#The%20Schools%20Beginnings.
27. Megan Ford, "Focus: A Brief History of Men in Nursing," *Nursing Times* (6 March 2019). nursingtimes.net/research-and-innovation/focus-a-brief-history-of-men-in-nursing-06-03-2019/, cdn.ps.emap.com/wp-content/uploads/sites/3/2019/03/010-011_NT_MAR19.pdf.

28. *See* "Francis Evelyn Windsor," *Canadian Great War Project*. canadiangreatwarproject.com/person.php?pid=99881/. In 1917 she married Edward Leacock, a brother of the writer Stephen Leacock. On her significant career as a pioneering doctor working with Indigenous People, and women and children in Calgary, see Laurie Meijer Drees, "Native Images: Reserve Hospitals in Southern Alberta, 1890 to 1930," *Native Studies Review* 9:1 (1993–94), 93–109. iportal.usask.ca/record/34111/.
29. Jill MacMicken-Wilson, "MacKenzie, Eliza (Elizabeth) Margaret," *Dictionary of Canadian Biography*, vol. 16, University of Toronto/Université Laval, 2003–. biographi.ca/en/bio/mackenzie_eliza_margaret_16E.html.
30. Andrew Macphail, *Official History of the Canadian Forces in the Great War 1914–19: The Medical Service* (National Defence, 1925), 222.
31. *See* Debbie Marshall, *Give Your Other Vote to the Sister: A Woman's Journey into the Great War* (University of Calgary Press, 2007).
32. Maude Abbott, "Lectures on the History of Nursing," *The Canadian Nurse* 19:3 (March 1923), 147–9. canadian-nurse.com/viewdocument/march-1923.
33. Linda J. Quiney, "Gendering Patriotism: Canadian Volunteer Nurses as the Female 'Soldiers' of the Great War,'" in Sarah Glassford and Amy Shaw, eds, *A Sisterhood of Suffering and Service: Women and Girls of Canada and Newfoundland During the First World War* (UBC Press, 2012), 107.
34. ———, "'Filling the Gaps': Canadian Voluntary Nurses, the 1917 Halifax Explosion, and the Influenza Epidemic of 1918," *Canadian Bulletin of Medical History*, 19:2 (2002), 352. doi.org/10.3138/cbmh.19.2.351.
35. Ibid., 357.
36. Lyn Macdonald, *The Roses of No Man's Land* (Penguin, 1980), 214.
37. Quiney, "Filling the Gaps," 357.
38. Ethel M. McCarthy, *Report on the Work of the CAMC Nursing Service with the BEF in France. Great War Accounts: Canadian Nurses*, Scarlett Finders, copyright by The National Archives WO222/2134. scarletfinders.co.uk/20.html.
39. Quiney, "Gendering," 117. There is a photograph of these women when they were serving at Pine Hill Convalescent Hospital in M.S. Hunt, ed., *Nova Scotia's Part in the Great War* (Nova Scotia Veteran Publishing, 1920), 424. Edith was a witness when Doull married Harry Christie Bauld in New Glasgow in 1922. She served as secretary treasurer of the Red Cross Society until 1939. Terry Bishop Stirling, "'Such Sights One

Will Never Forget': Newfoundland Women and Overseas Nursing in the First World War," in Sarah Glassford and Amy Shaw, eds, *A Sisterhood of Suffering and Service: Women and Girls of Canada and Newfoundland During the First World War* (UBC Press, 2012), 126–47.

40. Quiney, *Filling the Gaps*, 352, 354, 355. Glassford, *Mobilizing Mercy* (McGill-Queen's University Press, 2017), 99–101. Surprisingly, Quiney stated in "Assistant Angels: Canadian Voluntary Aid Detachment Nurses in the Great War" in 1998 that "approximately 500 Canadian VADs served "both at home and overseas" (p. 191).
41. Toman, *Sister Soldiers*, 68.
42. A. H., "The War," *The Canadian Nurse*, 11:1 (January 1915), 20. canadian-nurse.com/viewdocument/january-1915.
43. Jean Gunn, "The Service of Canadian Nurses and Voluntary Aids During the War," *Canadian Nurse* vol.15 (September 1919), 1975–79. canadian-nurse.com/viewdocument/september-1919.
44. Her name is often spelled "Veits," but the correct spelling is "Viets."

Chapter 1

45. Tim Cook, *At the Sharp End: Canadians Fighting the Great War 1914–1916* (Penguin, 2007), 54.
46. Mabel B. Clint, *Our Bit: Memories of War Service by a Canadian Nursing Sister* (Barwick, 1934), 11.
47. *See* Macphail, *Official History*, 222; Susan Mann, *Margaret Macdonald*, 75; Tim Cook, *Life Savers and Body Snatchers: Medical Care and the Struggle for Survival in the Great War* (Toronto, 2022), 29.
48. Adami, *War Story*, 235.
49. Clint, *Our Bit*, 13.
50. R. J. Manion, *A Surgeon in Arms* (McLelland, Goodchild & Stewart, 1918), 2. Manion was a physician in Fort William, Ontario, who joined the CAMC in 1915 and served overseas with the 21st Battalion. He supported conscription and was elected in 1917 as a Liberal Unionist, then served in the governments of Arthur Meighen and R. B. Bennett. Defeated in the 1935 election, he won a by-election in London and led the Conservative Party from 1938 but was defeated in 1940. The government appointed him director of civilian air raid defence.
51. George G. Nasmith, *On the Fringe of the Great Fight* (McLelland, Goodchild & Stewart, 1917), 7. Nasmith was Toronto's deputy health officer and a water purification and sanitation expert when the war broke out. He went overseas with the first contingent as commanding officer of

the Canadian Mobile Laboratory with the rank of lieutenant colonel, responsible for ensuring that the troops were provided with purified water. When the Germans launched chlorine gas at Ypres in 1915, he identified it and quickly devised the first gas masks that became part of the Allies' equipment.

52. Clint, *Our Bit*, 17.
53. Nasmith, *On the Fringe*, 8.
54. Clint, *Our Bit*, 17.
55. Ibid.
56. *The Globe*, May 25, 1916, quoted in Toman, *Sister Soldiers*, 17. Born at Pictou, Nova Scotia, Robert Rudolf was educated in England and Scotland and practised medicine in Edinburgh and India before settling in Toronto, where he served on the staffs of the General Hospital and the Hospital for Sick Children and also taught at the University of Toronto. He joined the CAMC and went overseas with the first contingent and served in No 2 CGH in France and later as consulting physician to the Canadian forces in England, with the rank of lieutenant colonel.
57. Nasmith, untitled article in the *Canadian Nurse* vol. 18 (January 1922), 39–40. canadian-nurse.com/viewdocument/january-1922; *The Globe*, May 25, 1916, quoted in Toman, *Sister Soldiers*, 17.
58. Susan Mann, *Margaret Macdonald*, 80.
59. Adami, *War Story*, 235.
60. For a good account of nursing in casualty clearing stations, see Christine E. Hallett, "Saving Lives on the Front Line," *History Today* 67:7 (July 2017), 24–35. historytoday.com/archive/saving-lives-front-line.
61. Ibid., 91.
62. The five hospital ships were HMHS *Araguaya*, HMHS *Essequibo*, HMHS *Letitia*, HMHS *Llandovery Castle* and HMHS *Neuralia*. Other ships that were not designated hospital ships but carried nurses were SS *Megantic*, SS *Royal George*, HMT *Tunisian* and HMT *Khyber*. HMHS *Goorkha* was a transport and hospital ship that carried seventeen nurses and 362 soldiers from Salonika to Malta when it struck a mine in October 1917, but there were no casualties.
63. McCarthy, "Report on the Work of the CAMC Nursing Service." R. C. Fetherstonhaugh, the historian of No. 3 CGH, claims that it was the "first of the universities of the empire to offer a medical unit, bearing its name, for service overseas. R. C. Fetherstonhaugh, *No. 3 General Hospital (McGill), 1914–1919* (Gazette Print, 1928), 6. That was true, but No. 2 CSH was the first Canadian hospital in the field.

64. Born in Hamilton, Ontario, Ethel Blanche Ridley earned a BA degree at the University of Toronto and trained at the New York Training School for Nurses. She served with the US army in the Philippines during the Spanish-American War, did medical missionary work in China, then returned to New York and was nursing at the Hospital for Ruptured and Cripples when she joined the CAMC at Valcartier in September 1914 as Macdonald's assistant. She served in hospitals in England and was awarded several decorations including the 1914 Star, the Royal Red Cross 1st Class, and the CBE. She subsequently returned to New York City and was director of nurses at the New York Orthopaedic Hospital until her retirement in 1942.
65. Harriet Graham letter, undated [December 3, 1914], published in the *Eastern Chronicle* (New Glasgow), December 24, 1914.
66. Ibid.
67. M. Leslie Newell, "'Led by the Spirit of Humanity': Canadian Military Nursing, 1914–1929," Unpublished MSc in Nursing Thesis, (University of Ottawa, 1996), 2, 58. dx.doi.org/10.20381/ruor-8193.
68. Clint, *Our Bit*, 32.
69. Graham letter, *Eastern Chronicle*, December 24, 1914.
70. Ibid.
71. Harriet Graham letter to New Glasgow Red Cross Society, February 22, 1915; published in the *Eastern Chronicle* (New Glasgow), March 19, 1915.
72. Adruenna Tupper to her mother, May 6, 1915, published in *Bridgewater Bulletin,* June 1, 1915. Tupper was serving in No. 2 Canadian Stationary Hospital at Le Trépport at the time.
73. The Royal Red Cross was introduced in 1883 to recognize nurses who showed exceptional devotion and competency in the performance of actual nursing duties over a continuous and long period or who had performed some very exceptional act of bravery and devotion at their post of duty. In December 1917 a bar was added to recognize further bravery or devotion to duty.
74. H. W. Hiltz letter to the secretary of Kingsport Red Cross Society, January 4, 1916, published in *Kentville Advertiser*, February 11, 1916.
75. James M. Cameron, *Pictonians in Arms: A Military History of Pictou County, Nova Scotia* (University of New Brunswick, 1969), 105.
76. Joseph Hayes, "Nova Scotia Medical Services in the Great War," in M. S. Hunt, *Nova Scotia's Part in the Great War* (Nova Scotia Veteran Publishing, 1920), 185.
77. Fetherstonhaugh, *No. 3 Canadian General Hospital*, 9.

78. It is often referred to as "Dannes-Camiers," but Dannes is the local train station.
79. Fetherstonhaugh, *No. 3 Canadian General Hospital*, 30.
80. Ibid., 40.
81. Ibid., 41–2.
82. Ibid., 40.
83. Ibid., 57, 61, 87.
84. Ibid., 148.
85. Ibid., 148–150.
86. Ibid.
87. Ibid., 62.
88. Andrew Beckett and Edward J. Harvey, "No. 3 Canadian General Hospital (McGill) in the Great War: Service and Sacrifice," *Canadian Journal of Surgery* 61:1 (2018), 8–12. doi.org/10.1503/cjs.012717. Next to Fetherstonhaugh's book, the best source of information on No. 3 CGH is the war diary of Clare Gass, which has been published with introduction and notes by Susan Mann as *The War Diary of Clare Gass, 1915–1918* (McGill-Queen's University Press, 2000). Also somewhat useful is Ross Hebb, *A Canadian Nurse in the Great War: The Diaries of Ruth Loggie, 1915–1916* (Nimbus Publishing, 2021). Loggie was a nurse from New Brunswick who served with Gass in No. 3 CGH.
89. Osler's son, Edward Revere Osler, enlisted in No. 3 CGH in February 1915, but when it moved to Boulogne, he transferred into the Royal Field Artillery with the rank of lieutenant and was killed in August 1917.
90. Beckett and Harvey, "No. 3 Canadian General Hospital," 10.
91. Barry Cahill, "STEWART, JOHN (1848–1933)," in *Dictionary of Canadian Biography,* vol. 16, University of Toronto/Université Laval, 2003–. biographi.ca/en/bio/stewart_john_1848_1933_16E.html.
92. Bernier and McAlister, "The Canadian Army Medical Corps Affair," 36.
93. With the exception of the Victoria General and St. Joseph's, hospitals in Nova Scotia offered two-year nurse training programs, but their graduates did not meet the same standards as those who completed a university-based three-year program.
94. "Other ranks" referred to orderlies and others who supported the work of the doctors and nurses. For No. 7 CSH's Nominal Roll of Officers, Non-Commissioned Officers and Men, see recherche-collection-search.bac-lac.gc.ca/eng/home/record?app=fonandcol&idnumber=5713998&ecopy=e011087862&wbdisable=false.
95. Hayes, "Nova Scotia Medical Services," 177–225.

96. Wilhelmina "Irene" Thompson's diary, undated, quoted in Stanley T. Spicer, *Ashore & Afloat* (Lancelot Press, 1993), 82.
97. Ibid., 83.
98. Curiously, Carruthers was listed as a major on No. 9 CSH's nominal roll, but he actually joined the 64th Battalion as medical officer and went to England in March 1916. When it was disbanded in December 1917, he was promoted to lieutenant colonel in command of Woodcote Park Military Convalescent Hospital, Epsom, the largest convalescent hospital in England. He fell ill with neurasthenia in September 1918, perhaps because his wife had died in August, and he was invalided in 1919 to Ste Anne de Bellevue Military Hospital in Montreal.
99. Cameron, *For the People*, 161.
100. Ibid. The other six were Emma Barry, Florence Kelly, Nellie King, Mary McGrath, Catherine Shea and Mary Walsh. *No. 9 Stationary Hospital Nominal Roll of Officers, Nursing Sisters, Non-Commissioned Officers and Men.* Canadian Expeditionary Force (Canadian Expeditionary Force, 1917). n2t.net/ark:/69429/m0z892806k1r.
101. His name on his attestation document is given as "McLeod," but the family spelled it as "MacLeod."
102. Bruce MacDonald, "Sgt. Horace Goddard MacMillan: A 'Stationary Hospital' Soldier's Story," *First World War Veterans of Guysborough County.* guysboroughgreatwarveterans.blogspot.com/2013/05/sgt-horace-goddard-macmillan-stationary.html.
103. Cameron, *For the People*, 161.
104. In October 1917, it was redesignated No. 12 Canadian General Hospital.
105. Kendall also served as lieutenant governor of Nova Scotia from 1942 to 1947, the oldest person ever to hold the office. His brother, Arthur Kendall, was also a physician and a Liberal politician who represented Cape Breton County in the House of Assembly from 1897 to 1900 and 1904 to 1911 and in the House of Commons from 1900 to 1904.
106. Lyndsay Rosenthal, "Venus in the Trenches: The Treatment of Venereal Disease in the Canadian Expeditionary Force, 1914–1919," *Theses and Dissertations (Comprehensive)*. 2107. (Wilfrid Laurier University, 2018), 1–2. scholars.wlu.ca/etd/2107.
107. Mark G. McGowan, "Harvesting the 'Red Vineyard': Catholic Religious Culture in the Canadian Expeditionary Force, 1914–1919," *Canadian Catholic Historical Association Historical Studies* 64 (1998), 51–2, 61–4. cchahistory.ca/journal/CCHA1998/McGowan.htm.
108. Cameron, *For the People*, 161, 163.
109. Rosenthal, "Venus in the Trenches," 124–5.

110. Ibid., 157–8. Scott Matheson, "In the Dust You Will Prevail: The Mobilization of Acadia, Dalhousie, Mount Allison, and St. Francis Xavier Universities, 1914–1918" Saint Mary's University, 2010. library2.smu.ca/xmlui/handle/01/23728.

Chapter 2

111. Jean-Robert Bernier and Vivian C. McAlister, "The Canadian Army Medical Corps Affair of 1916 and Surgeon General Guy Carleton Jones," *Canadian Journal of Surgery* 61:2 (April 2018), 85–87. doi.org/10.1503/cjs.003818.
112. Clint, *Our Bit*, 54.
113. Adami, *War Story*, 260.
114. Christine E. Hallett, *Veiled Warriors: Allied Nurses of the First World War* (Oxford University Press, 2014), 136.
115. Adami, *War Story*, 259–60.
116. Ibid., 261–2.
117. Cynthia Toman, "'A Loyal Body of Empire Citizens': Military Nurses and Identity at Lemnos and Salonika, 1915–17," in Jayne Elliott, Meryn Stuart and Cynthia Toman, *Place and Practice in Canadian Nursing History* (UBC Press, 2008), 19.
118. Clint, *Our Bit*, 63, 65–81.
119. Ibid., 63.
120. Suzanna Wagner, "Many Places, Many Problems: Canadian First War Military Nursing Sisters in the Mediterranean" Master's Thesis, University of Alberta, 2020. doi.org/10.7939/r3-56vz-9t73.
121. Katherine Wilson-Simmie, *Lights Out! The Memoirs of Nursing Sister Kate Wilson, Canadian Army Medical Corps 1915–1917* (CEF Books, 2004), 62–3.
122. Adami, *War Story*, 263.
123. Wilson, *Lights Out*, 161.
124. *Nova Scotia Legislature Debates and Proceedings*, April 13, 2018, Resolution 1305, p. 4075; nslegislature.ca/legislative-business/hansard-debates/assembly-63-session-1/house_18apr13#HPage4075.
125. Wagner, "Many Places," 109.
126. Clint, *Our Bit*, 80.
127. Project Team, First World War Poetry Digital Archive. "53855: The Sisters Buried at Lemnos." University of Oxford, May 1, 2024. doi.org/10.25446/oxford.25732062.v1.

128. J. J. Mackenzie, *Number 4 Canadian Hospital: The Letters of Professor J. J. Mackenzie from the Salonika Front* (Macmillan, 1933).
129. Nursing Sister C.I.S. [pseud.], "Hospital Ship Life in the Mediterranean," *The Canadian Nurse* vol.18 (January 1922), 31–2. canadian-nurse.com/viewdocument/january-1922. Mackenzie, *Number 4*, 41.
130. Mackenzie, *Number 4*, 51.
131. Ibid., 55–6, 73–4.
132. Gerald W. L. Nicholson, *Canada's Nursing Sisters* (Samuel Stevens, 1975), 497.
133. "Davis, Lena Aloa," *The Canadian Letters & Images Project*, Vancouver Island University. canadianletters.ca/collections/all/collection/67329/. "Lena Aloa Davis," canadiangreatwarproject.com/person.php?pid=69057.
134. Wagner, "Many Places," 71.
135. Mackenzie, *Number 4*, 69.
136. Ibid., 55, 92–95, 105, 114, 148, 151, 156.
137. Ibid., 223. The White Tower was a proud landmark because it was a fortress constructed by the Venetians in the fifteenth century to protect Salonika from attack.
138. Ibid., 158, 148.
139. Wagner, "Many Places," 76.
140. Ibid., 99, 111–12.
141. Ibid., 43, 78. *See* Toman, "A Loyal Body," 18.
142. Wagner, "Many Places," 43.
143. Ibid., 31.
144. Ibid., 264, 266–7.

Chapter 3

145. David Mossman, *Going Over: A Nova Scotia Soldier in World War I* (Pottersfield Press, 2014), 50.
146. *Morning Chronicle*, June 19, 1918.
147. Thompson's diary, 84.
148. Chryssa N. McAlister, Allan E. Marble and T. Jock Murray, "The 1917 Halifax Explosion: The First Coordinated Local Civilian Medical Response to Disaster in Canada," *Canadian Journal of Surgery* 60:6 (2017): 372–4. doi.org/10.1503/cjs.016317.
149. Sharon Adams, "The Halifax Explosion," *Legion Magazine*, December 13, 2017. legionmagazine.com/features/halifax-explosion/.

150. Wendy Elliott, "Nova Scotian Nurses Among the Unsung Heroes of the First World War," *Halifax Chronicle Herald*, published October 2, 2014, last updated on September 30, 2017. saltwire.com/atlantic-canada/nova-scotian-nurses-among-the-unsung-heroes-of-the-first-world-war-51724. *See* Joyce Glasner, "On the Frontlines of Disaster," *Canada's History* (December 2017–January 2018). canadashistory.ca/explore/transportation/on-the-frontlines-of-disaster. On the DeWitts, see Randall House, "From Sanitation to the Sanatorium: The Doctors DeWitt and Their Sixty Years of Service," *Randall Posts*, August 6, 2014. randallposts.wordpress.com/2014/08/06/from-sanitation-to-the-sanatorium-the-doctors-dewitt-and-their-sixty-years-of-service/.
151. Quoted in Laura M. MacDonald, *Curse of the Narrows: The Halifax Explosion 1917* (HarperCollins, 2005): 134. *See* Mark Osborne Humphries, "BELL, FREDERICK McKELVEY," in *Dictionary of Canadian Biography*, vol. 16, University of Toronto/Université Laval, 2003–). biographi.ca/en/bio/bell_frederick_mckelvey_16E.html.
152. Gilbert Tucker, *The Naval Service of Canada: Its Official History* (National Defence, 1952): 233.
153. The naval hospital's building "remained standing with its walls and roof intact," but its condition "was such that the staff and cadets had to be moved, and they were sent to Kingston, Ontario, although it continued to operate." Formerly the residence of the British admiral commanding the Halifax naval base, Admiralty House had been taken over from the Royal Navy by the Canadian government in 1905 when it took over the Halifax Dockyard. When the war broke out, it served as a naval hospital until being damaged during the explosion. Despite having its roof, ceilings and walls collapsed and its windows blown out, hospital staff, many of whom who had been injured, treated injured people in the hours after the explosion. After repairs, it was used by the Massachusetts-Halifax Relief Commission as a public health facility for the area.
154. Thomas Raddall, *In My Time: A Memoir* (McLelland and Stewart, 1976): 36.
155. St Mary's College was a Catholic boys' school on Grafton Street.
156. The Claytons contributed their home in nearby Rockingham to the Military Hospitals Commission to be used as a convalescent hospital, and its first patients were seventeen Jamaican soldiers who had arrived in Halifax en route to England in the winter of 1915–16 because their feet had been seriously frozen. According to a report in the *Canadian Medical Journal*, it was the "first Canadian hospital devoted exclusively to vocational training." *Canadian Medical Journal* 6:10 (October 1916):

925–6. *See* Brian Douglas Tennyson, *Nova Scotia at War 1914–1919* (Nimbus Publishing, 2017): 115-16. The Claytons' only son, Edward, served as a captain in the 85th Battalion and was killed at Passchendaele in October 1917. Two months later the Claytons' clothing factory, the largest in Eastern Canada, situated on what is now the site of Scotia Square, was destroyed in the Halifax explosion.

157. Raddall, *In My Time.*
158. Harry Chapman, *In the Wake of the Alderney: Dartmouth, Nova Scotia, 1750–2000* (Dartmouth Historical Association, 2001), 198, 201.
159. For a good contemporary account of the explosion's impact on Dartmouth, see Rev. J. A. McGlashen, minister of Stairs Memorial Church, in the *Progress-Enterprise* (Lunenburg), February 13, 1918.
160. *Sydney Record*, undated, reprinted in the *Daily News* (Truro), December 24, 1917. *See* the *CMA Journal* vol. 8 (February 1918), 169. For a report on the role of physicians in the crisis, see the *CMA Journal* vol. 8 (January 1918), 59–62.
161. Robert Laird Borden, *Robert Laird Borden: His Memoirs, Volume 2*, ed. Henry Borden (McGill-Queen's University Press, 1938), 764.
162. Quoted in Laura M. MacDonald, *Curse of the Narrows: The Halifax Explosion 1917* (HarperCollins, 2005), 105.
163. John Griffith Armstrong, *The Halifax Explosion and the Royal Canadian Navy: Inquiry and Intrigue* (UBC Press, 2002), 97. MacDonald, *Curse of the Narrows*, 206.
164. Dr. Allan Marble, "Halifax Was Plunged into Gloom: The Impact of the Spanish Influenza Pandemic on Nova Scotia," *Journal of the Royal Nova Scotia History Society* vol. 22 (2019), 25. Among the nurses who served in Boston were Judy Cadegan, Hilda Chisholm, Jessie Chisholm, Gertrude Crosby, Mary Duffie, Nora Duncanson, Georgina and Winnifred Flemming, Lottie Flick, Annie Gilmour, H. M. Godfrey, Christine McInnis, Dorothy Merlin, Carrie Mitchell, Greta Ogle, Ethel Redmond, Ethel Taylor and Mary Tompkins.

Chapter 4

165. Delaney Beck, "Bluebirds, Bombings, and Battle: Shell Shock in Maritime Nursing Sisters of the First World War" MA thesis (Saint Mary's University, 2001), 68. library2.smu.ca/handle/01/29960.

166. *War Diary of No. 1 Canadian General Hospital*, volume 18:5 (May 19, 1918), 6. recherche-collection-search.bac-lac.gc.ca/eng/home/record?idnumber=2005096&app=fonandcol&q=war%20diaries%20general%20hospital&ecopy=e001513825. Canadian Expeditionary Force Research Group, "No.1 Canadian General Hospital in the Great War." Units Great War, CEFRG.ca. cefrg.ca/no-1-canadian-general-hospital/. *See* Helen Dore Boylston, *Sister: The War Diary of a Nurse* (Eves Washburn, 1927), 54, 55; and Thompson's diary, 85.
167. Beck, "Bluebirds," 68.
168. Bruce MacDonald, "Lieutenant Charlotte 'Lottie' Urquhart—A Military Medal Nursing Sister's Story," *First World War Veterans of Guysborough County*, May 31, 2018. guysboroughgreatwarveterans.blogspot.com/2018/05/lieutenant-charlotte-lottie-urquharta.html.
169. Thompson's diary, 85.
170. Stewart had been appointed surgical consultant to hospitals in England.
171. Thompson's diary, 84.
172. Ibid., 85.
173. Jill Stewart, "The First Canadian Nurses Killed by Enemy Action During the First World War," *Western Front Association*. westernfrontassociation.com/world-war-i-articles/the-first-canadian-nurses-killed-by-enemy-action-during-the-first-world-war/.
174. T. Robert Fowler, "The Canadian Nursing Service and the British War Office: The Debate Over Awarding the Military Cross, 1918," *Canadian Military History* 14:4 (2005), 36. scholars.wlu.ca/cmh/vol14/iss4/4/.
175. *No. 3 CSH War Diary*. Adami's figures are two surgeons, three nurses, four patients and thirteen orderlies. Adami, *War Story*, 239. *cf.* Hallett, *Veiled Warriors*, 237.
176. Edith Campbell came from a prominent medical family in Montreal with close ties to Sir William Osler. *See* Michael Bliss, *William Osler: A Life in Medicine* (Oxford University Press, 1999), 428–31. She had previously served as the first matron of the DCRC before being transferred to No. 1 CGH, No. 8 CGH, and finally No. 3 CSH.
177. *See* Fowler, "Canadian Nursing Service," 31–42.
178. Hallett, *Veiled Warriors*, 244.
179. Tim Cook, *Lifesavers and Body Snatchers: Medical Care and the Struggle for Survival in the Great War* (Penguin Canada, 2022), 426.
180. Macphail, *Official History*, 24. He also gave the figure as thirty-eight on page 245, presumably an error.
181. "Report of the Unveiling Ceremony of the Memorial to the Canadian Nursing Sisters," *Canadian Nurse* vol. 22 (October 1926), 537–45. canadian-nurse.com/viewdocument/october-1926.

182. Dianne Dodd, "Canadian Military Nurse Deaths in the First World War," *Canadian Bulletin of Medical History* 34:2 (Fall 2017), 327. doi.org/10.3138/cbmh.34.2.131-30072014. *See* "Nurse Bertha Bartlett," Trail of the Caribou group, *Facebook*. facebook.com/media/set/?set=a.31429830224897328&type=3&comment_id=3144611172326917&reply_comment_id=3148073331980701&paipv=0&eav=Afb3Xvyvc-U8522uHd2sibZBEO9Zhr6viV2zoVIKWRRdrbxYyMVvL8olL-33MyRp5GpFk&_rdr/. Peter Grant, "Dorothy Pearson Twist," *Spanish Influenza in Victoria, Canada, 1918–1920*. spanishfluvictoriabc.com/dorothy-pearson-twist/. The number of other ranks who died was 532. *See* Nic Hume, "Remembrance: In Quiet Cobble Hill, Cenotaph Honours Daughter Who Fell in First World War," *Vancouver Sun* (November 10, 1921). vancouversun.com/news/local-news/remembrance-in-quiet-cobble-hill-cenotaph-honours-daughter-who-fell-in-first-world-war/.
183. Macphail, *Official History*, 219. Desmond Morton, *When Your Number's Up: The Canadian Soldier in the First World War* (Random House, 1993), 181.
184. Nicholson, *Canada's Nursing Sisters*, 98–9. MacPhail's figures were 328 decorations, 33 Royal Red Crosses, 169 mentions in dispatches, and 76 brought to the notice of the Secretary of State for War. Fifty others received foreign honours. Macphail, *Official History,* 224–5. The CAMC Nursing Service's numbers were different again. *cf.* Ethel McCarthy, "Report on the Work of the CAMC Nursing Service."
185. "The Nursing Sisters' Memorial," Veterans Affairs Canada. veterans.gc.ca/en/remembrance/memorials/canada/nurses-memorial.
186. It included 1,513 nurses, 43 of whom were Canadians. "The Sisters Window for the Sisters," York Minster, Chapter of York. yorkminster.org/discover/stories/story/the-sisters-window-for-the-sisters/.
187. Sarah Glassford, "Soldiering On After the Armistice: Health, Work and Family in the Lives of Some Canadian Army Medical Corps Nurse Veterans," *Canadian Military History* 32:1 (2003), 1–24. scholars.wlu.ca/cmh/vol32/iss1/21/.

Database

188. Where one or both parents are marked as "deceased," it indicates the parent(s) died before the nurse's enlistment, as recorded on the Officers' Declaration Paper.
189. Her CEF service file and marriage certificate give her middle name as Hazen, but all other official records give it as Hazel.

190. The Harvard Surgical Unit originated in the spring of 1915 to provide medical services to the British and French in the war. Instruments and supplies were organized through the Massachusetts General and two other hospitals. It went overseas in March 1915 and began by providing staffing at the American Ambulance Hospital in Paris, then became the Harvard Surgical Unit in November 1916, which functioned as an integral part of the British army as the British government granted its members commissioned rank in the Royal Army Medical Corps, although it was officially a neutral organization and travelled under the auspices of the Red Cross. It was stationed at the RAMC No. 22 General Hospital at Camiers.
191. *The Morning Chronicle* (Halifax), December 13, 1917. She is not listed on the Canadian Soldiers database because she was a Royal Canadian Navy nurse. *The Canadian Navy List for July, 1919*, Department of the Naval Service (Ottawa, 1919), 73. navalandmilitarymuseum.org/wp-content/uploads/2019/06/CFB-Esquimalt-Museum-Navy-List-1919-July-Vol-2.pdf.
192. Her middle name is sometimes spelled "Squaire," but she spelled it "Squair."
193. Tina Comeau, "'Sara Corning's Life Reads Like One of Legend': Memorial Park Dedicated in Yarmouth in her Honour," *Tri-County Vanguard*, September 23, 2025. saltwire.com/nova-scotia/tri-county-vangaurd/sara-cornings-life-reads-like-one-of-legend-memorial-park-dedicated-in-yarmouth-in-her-honour/.
194. See his army service record and his biography at "Robert Cray Simpson," Obituaries, Echovita. echovita.com/ca/obituaries/ab/sherwood-park/robert-cray-simpson-16073372.
195. "George S. & Jessie Haddon House," Heritage Burnaby. search.heritageburnaby.ca/link/landmark508/.
196. "1931 Census of Canada," Ancestry.ca. ancestry.ca/search/collections/62640/records/10222396?tid=&pid=&queryId=a31e9a88-c086-4573-bdfd-b97b310f01a3&_phsrc=RWd825&_phstart=successSource/.
197. In 1926 she claimed that her date of birth was 1887.
198. He represented Cape Breton South and Richmond from 1921 to 1925, then was appointed a judge in the Nova Scotia Supreme Court but resigned in 1949 and was elected in Inverness-Richmond, retiring in 1953.
199. Stephens, *Remembering Nurses*, 42.
200. James Percy McNaughton's first wife, Etta Peppett, the daughter of a prominent North Sydney businessman, had died in 1915, leaving him with three children. ancestry.com/genealogy/records/james-percy-mcnaughton-24-kofm3/.

201. Lynn Curwin, "Truro Editor and Doctor Among the First to Help Following Halifax Explosion," *PNI Atlantic*, published July 20, 2017. Updated September 30, 2017. saltwire.com/atlantic-canada/truro-editor-and-doctor-among-the-first-to-help-following-halifax-explosion-153297/.
202. "Evangeline Eaton," Ancestry.ca. ancestry.ca/search/collections/2442/records/73317666/.
203. "Nurses of World War I.... A Legacy of Compassion and Caring," Wartime Heritage Association. wartimeheritage.com/storyarchive1/story_nurses_wwi.htm.
204. General Douglas MacArthur, "General Orders No. 3," War Department, February 22, 1932; and Fred L. Borch, "A Heart of Purple: The Story of American's Oldest Military Decoration and Some of Its Recipients," *Prologue* vol. 44:4 (Winter 2012), 18. archives.gov/publications/prologue/2012/winter/heart-of-purple.
205. When she joined the CAMCNS, she gave her name as "Edith Lilian Morrow Fraser," but she did not include "Lilian" in her documents.
206. The Canadian Great War Project website claims that she died in 1939, but according to the 1953 Canadian Voters list, she was nursing in Arichat, Richmond County. canadiangreatwarproject.com/person.php?pid=88594/.
207. "Nursing Sister Florence Amelia Fraser," Find a Grave. findagrave.com/memorial/270997156/florence-a-fraser#source/.
208. "Nursing Sister Florence Mathilda Fraser," Find a Grave. findagrave.com/memorial/284747771/florence-mathilda-fraser/.
209. *Nurses' Directory* 1923–24, 33.
210. Obituaries, *Montreal Gazette*, October 23, 1948.
211. "Margaret A. Fraser," Antigonish Heritage Museum, Antigonish Heritage Society. antigonishheritage.ca/margaret-a-fraser/; "Margaret Ann 'Maggie A' Fraser," Ancestry.ca, ancestry.ca/family-tree/person/tree/195971299/person/352563465544/facts.
212. "Lieutenant Gertrude Frazee," Canadian Great War Project. canadiangreatwarproject.com/person.php?pid=85817.
213. They married in June 1904, but he died by suicide in September 1905. *Saint John's Evening Telegram*, September 15, 1905. "William Syme Frew," Find a Grave, findagrave.com/memorial/202551786/william-syme-frew/; FamilySearch, familysearch.org/ark:/61903/1:1:4KHD-Y6PZ/; and "Frances Maitland Blair (1879–1975)," WikiTree, wikitree.com/wiki/Blair-13548.
214. "Mary Sophia (Fulton) Street (1889–1980)," WikiTree. wikitree.com/wiki/Fulton-3683.

215. "Vernon Serves: Remembering the Men & Women Who Have Served Canada in War and Peace," Greater Vernon Museum & Archives. vernonmuseum.ca/vernon-serves/.
216. *London Gazette* (29 June 1923), 4516; Canadian Great War Project. canadiangreatwarproject.com/person.php?pid=93941.
217. "Sarah Jane (Lillywhite) Gilbert (1858–1937)," WikiTree. wikitree.com/wiki/Lillywhite-36.
218. *Calgary Herald*, April 27, 1972; "Lt NS Phyllis Nora Gilbert," Find a Grave; findagrave.com/memorial/137456552/phyllis-nora-gilbert/.
219. Western Hospital School of Nursing in London, Ontario, amalgamated with the Montreal General Hospital in 1924, becoming the Western Division of the Montreal General Hospital.
220. Anon., "Ship Hector Passenger Descendents: Harriet Graham MacDonald," *PNI Atlantic News*, June 7, 2023. saltwire.com/atlantic-canada/ship-hector-passenger-descendents-harriet-graham-macdonald-100861127.
221. There is no official record of her date of birth, but an undated certification document in the Nova Scotia Archives declares that she was born in 1885, and this was the date she gave when she joined the CAMCNS. Her tombstone claims, however, that she was born in 1880. "Jean Augusta Harrison," Ancestry.ca. ancestry.ca/family-tree/person/tree/76439147/person/44341694324/facts.
222. "Tomlinson Jean Augusta (Harrison) WWI Veteran," Ancestry.ca. ancestry.ca/mediaui-viewer/tree/76439147/person/44341694324/media/deb87c14-44c8-4018-ab5d-d2ff70311641.
223. *Nurses' Directory* (1924), 25, 26; Nova Scotia Archives.
224. "We Remember John Ross, or Jonathan Howe," Lives of the First World War, Imperial War Museums. livesofthefirstworldwar.iwm.org.uk/lifestory/1986465/,
225. Her mother's maiden name was Langille, and she was the widow of Henry Dauphiney when she married Silas Hubley, who was Jennie's father.
226. Thomas Daigle, "Beauty out of Pain: Canadian Soldiers' Embroidery Was Therapy for the Scars of War," *CBC World*, November 9, 2018. cbc.ca/news/world/first-world-war-soldiers-altar-cloth-embroidery-1.4895370; See also, Maev Kennedy, "First World War Altar Frontal Back at St. Paul's Cathedral," *The Guardian*, August 1, 2014. theguardian.com/world/2014/aug/01/first-world-war-altar-frontal-st-pauls-cathedral.

227. Jane A. Delano, "The Red Cross: In Charge of," *The American Journal of Nursing* vol. 18:2 (November 1917), 124. journals.lww.com/ajnonline/citation/1917/11000/in_charge_of.12.aspx.
228. The Halifax Infirmary functioned as the city's Roman Catholic hospital until it was taken over by the provincial government in 1973. The building was closed when the present Halifax Infirmary on Summer Street opened in 1998.
229. "Nova Scotia Births, Marriages, and Deaths," Nova Scotia Archives. archives.novascotia.ca/vital-statistics/death/?ID=150129.
230. "Nursing Sister Myrtle Margaret Hunt," Canadian Virtual War Memorial. veterans.gc.ca/en/remembrance/memorials/canadian-virtual-war-memorial/detail/2755313?Myrtle%20Margaret%20Hunt.
231. Wendy Elliott, "Meet Jessie Brown Jaggard, Wolfville's Unsung War Hero," *Halifax Chronicle Herald*, September 29, 2019.
232. Robyn-Rose May, *Bluebirds at War: Canada's Fallen Nursing Sisters of the First World War* (Double Dagger Books, 2023), 19.
233. Ibid., 45.
234. "Case H00516: Request to Include 144 Pleasant Street, Dartmouth, Dartmouth, in the Registry of Heritage Property for the Halifax Regional Municipality," Halifax Heritage Advisory Committee, May 25, 2022. cdn.halifax.ca/sites/default/files/documents/city-hall/boards-committees-commissions/220525hac911.pdf.
235. *See* Laura Fraser, "'Remember That I Love You': A Soldier's Letters to His Sweetheart," *CBC News*. newsinteractives.cbc.ca/longform/remember-that-i-love-you-a-soldiers-letters-to-his-sweetheart/.
236. Morin-Pelletier, "At Peace with the Germans," 197.
237. Dorothy P. Cotton, daughter of Brigadier General William Cotton, was a graduate of the Royal Victoria Hospital in Montreal and served in No. 3 CGH until being sent to Russia as part of a group of thirty-seven doctors, nurses, orderlies and ten volunteers sent to support the Petrograd (formerly St. Petersburg) Hospital, then under Anglo-Russian direction. After being recalled to England, she returned to Petrograd in 1917 and witnessed the Russian Revolution. When she returned to England, she was appointed matron of an officers' hospital until 1918, when she was transferred to the Camp Hill Hospital in Halifax in 1918. She was demobilized in 1919, having received the British War Medal and the Victory Medal. A year later she was appointed to lead a nursing mission to establish a training school for nurses at Cotzea Hospital in Romania. She later worked briefly at the Rockefeller Institute in Paris (1921–22) until moving to Saskatchewan where she was a public health nurse with the VON. *See* Hallett, *Veiled Warriors*, 110–12.

238. 1911 Canadian Census.
239. "Adriana Robertson Layton," First World War Personnel Records Database, Library and Archives Canada, 23-7. recherche-collection-search.bac-lac.gc.ca/eng/home/record?app=pffww&idnumber=522025&ecopy=453122a.
240. "Hants County Faces," Captured in Time. novascotianfaces.weebly.com/hants-et.html, novascotianfaces.weebly.com/hants-lay.html.
241. Although she was a francophone, she signed documents as "Mary," not "Marie."
242. *Nurses' Directory*, 1923–24, 32.
243. *Nurses' Directory*, 1924–25, 27.
244. When she joined the CAMC, she gave her date of birth as 1893, but a delayed registration of birth issued in 1951 declared that she was born in 1892.
245. *Nurses' Directory*, 1923–24, 34.
246. "Nursing Sister Olla Dell Lester Hare," Find a Grave. findagrave.com/memorial/268689087/olla_dell-hare/.
247. *Nurses' Directory*, 1923–24, 32.
248. *Nurses' Directory*, 1924–25, 27.
249. Canadian nursing students seeking maternity training were sent to Wesson Maternity Hospital in Springfield, Massachusetts, until 1916 when the Montreal General Hospital introduced such courses. It was not until 1922 that Halifax's Grace Maternity Hospital, founded in 1906 by the Salvation Army as a residential maternity hospital for unmarried women, was recognized by the Halifax Medical Association, and Dalhousie University offered both the land and the money to build it. Although affiliated as a teaching hospital with Dalhousie University's Department of Pediatrics, it was the only independent maternity hospital in Canada until 1992. It was replaced by the Izaak Walton Killam-Grace Health Centre for Children, Women and Families (now known as the IWK Health Centre).
250. Clyde F. Macdonald, *Faithful Services in WWI and WWII: Veterans of Sunny Brae, Pictou County* (New Glasgow, 2001), 125.
251. *Nurses' Directory*, 1923–24, 34. Her death certificate states that she had lived in Sydney since 1944.
252. "A Correction," *Star-Phoenix* (Saskatoon), April 22, 1919, p. 4. newspapers.com/article/star-phoenix/61920872/. "William Cameron Macintosh OBE (1894–1976)," WikiTree. wikitree.com/wiki/Macintosh-1068.

253. "Helen Catherine MacDonald," Ancestry.ca. ancestors.familysearch.org/en/G8CF-TFP/helen-catherine-macdonald-1886-1965.
254. "William Smith Beattie," Ancestry.ca. ancestry.ca/search/collections/60527/records/2494548/.
255. Gloria (Webb) Stephens, "1917—The Halifax Explosion and the VG Hospital," Nova Scotia Museum of Health Care, Association of Health Sciences Archives and Museums of Nova Scotia. novascotiamuseumofhealthcare.ca/resources/articles/.
256. "Jessie MacDonald," Antigonish Heritage Museum, Antigonish Heritage Society. antigonishheritage.ca/jessie-macdonald/.
257. "Nova Scotia Births, Marriages, and Deaths," Nova Scotia Archives. archives.novascotia.ca/vital-statistics/death/?ID=507298.
258. Her name is given on her attestation document as "Marguerite," but she signed her name "Margaret."
259. She was also loosely related to Sir John Thompson, a former premier of Nova Scotia, Minister of Justice and briefly Prime Minister of Canada, through her uncle Joseph Chisholm's wife, Frances Affleck, whose sister was Thompson's wife. Mann, *Margaret Macdonald,* 17.
260. Alexandra Minna Stern, ""The Public Health Service in the Panama Canal: A Forgotten Chapter of US Public Health," *Public Health Chronicles*, 120:6 (November–December 2005), 675–79. doi.org/10.1177/003335490512000616.
261. Allan Marble, "Hail to the Matron-in-Chief: Nova Scotian Margaret Clotilde MacDonald Led the Canadian Nursing Corps During First World War," *Vignettes*, Medical History Society of Nova Scotia, August 15, 2019. medicalhistoryns.com/vignettes/14-recent/337-hail-to-the-matron-in-chief-nova-scotian-margaret-clotilde-macdonald-led-the-canadian-nursing-corps-during-first-world-war.
262. "Margaret Katherine MacDonald," Find a Grave. findagrave.com/memorial/244320684/margaret-katherine-macdonald/.
263. *Nurses' Directory*, 1924–25, 27.
264. Her name is given on her attestation document as "Marguerite," but she signed her name "Margaret."
265. This information is based on Catherine MacGillivray's article, "Public Health Education in Antigonish County," *Old Train Station News* (Antigonish Heritage Museum), 52 (June 2013). antigonishheritage.ca/newsletter/.
266. "Nursing Sister Flora MacDougall," Find a Grave. findagrave.com/memorial/229406168/flora-macdougall/.

267. Anon, "Gone But Not Forgotten—Part 2: Sister Nurse Florence Louisa MacInnes and the Great War," Halifax Blogs: Local History (blog), Halifax Public Libraries, November 7, 2023. halifaxpubliclibraries.ca/blogs/post/gone-but-not-forgotten-part-2-sister-nurse-florence-louisa-macinnes-and-the-great-war/.
268. "George Cardno Edward," Commonwealth War Graves. cwgc.org/find-records/find-war-dead/casualty-details/2785983/george-cardno-edward/.
269. Mullins, *Some Liverpool Chronicles*, 145–6.
270. "Municipal Park Opened in Alberta in Honour of Big Island Woman," *Eastern Chronicle*, October 13, 1966; "Elizabeth I. Young," Ancestry.ca. ancestry.ca/mediaui-viewer/collection/1030/tree/26751574/person/12572331406/media/E85A479D-0808-baco-6760f61a77658?_phsrc=zdc1952&_phstay=successsource/.
271. For a detailed account of the Battle at Courcelette written by an officer who was there, see Robert Clements, *Merry Hell: The Story of the 25th Battalion (Nova Scotia Regiment)* (University of Toronto Press, 2013), 154–8.
272. Anne Gafiuk, "Jessie Margaret MacLeod C4169," WWII Canadian Women's Project. wwiicdnwomensproject.org/nurse/Jessie%20Margaret-MacLeod.html.
273. Maureen Duffus, *Battlefront Nurses in WW I* (Town and Gown Press, 2009).
274. Her actual date of birth is uncertain. Her death certificate said she was born in 1878, but in 1928 she submitted an affidavit to the provincial government declaring that she was born in 1888. Nova Scotia Births, Marriages, and Deaths, Nova Scotia Archives. archives.novascotia.ca/vital-statistics/birth/?ID=168511. The 1911 Canadian census stated that she was born in 1885.
275. Delano, "The Red Cross," 124. It is possible that this is not the same person.
276. *Advertiser* (Kentville), August 18, 1916.
277. His date of birth was given as "1890" in both the 1901 and 1911 censuses.
278. Her name is spelled "Katherine" on her death certificate.
279. Her surname is spelled "Paton" in all documents, including the 1901 and 1911 Canadian censuses, except the Nova Scotia Archives, where it is spelled "Patton."
280. In the 1920 US federal census, she claimed that she was born in Rhode Island.

281. "Mary Agnes Porter," Ancestry.ca. ancestors.familysearch.org/en/KNZ9-V9L/mary-agnes-porter-1869-1964/.
282. "Spencer in the Quebec, Canada, Vital and Church Records (Drouin Collection), 1621–1968," Ancestry.ca. ancestry.ca/discoveryui-content/view/29955339:1091. On Joseph William Spencer's background, see Greg Mercer, "Haunted by Memories of Cambridge's Coombe Orphanage," *Waterloo Region Record* (September 26, 2015); therecord.com/news/waterloo-region/haunted-by-memories-of-cambridges-coombe-orphanage/article_1376ebf8-dedd-5852-aaa7-5ce3cd7a7264.html
283. She may actually have been born in 1873.
284. "Memorable Manitobans: Annie Simpson Rathbone (1879–1953)"; Manitoba Historical Society Archives. mhs.mb.ca/docs/people/rathbone_as.shtml.
285. Elizabeth Service, *The Contributions of the Service Family to Sustainable Health Care in Sichuan* (Ottawa, 2021). library.vicu.utoronto.ca/exhibitions/vic_in_china/sections/missionaries_and_mission_stations/attachments/service_family_paper_april_2021.pdf.
286. Much of this information is from "Winnipeg General Hospital School of Nursing, Class of 1917," Health Sciences Centre Winnipeg Archives. hscarchives.com/winnipeg-general-hospital-school-of-nursing-class-of-1917.
287. The Boston Floating Hospital originated in 1894 as a rented excursion boat towed around Boston Harbour to give indigent mothers and their sick babies relief from the summer heat. It now operates in buildings and is an infant and childcare pediatric teaching institution. *See* "A History of the Boston Floating Hospital," *Pediatrics* 19:4 (1957), 629–38. doi.org/10.1542/peds.19.4.629.
288. *Nurses' Directory* 1923–24, 35.
289. It seems impossible to accurately determine her date of birth. She appears to have been born in 1869, but her parents married in about 1850. When she joined the CAMCNS, she claimed to have been born in 1878. Her tombstone says she was born in 1869.
290. "Nursing Sister Rev. Edith Alexandra Suzanne Murray Thompson," Find a Grave. findagrave.com/memorial/113361120/edith_alexandra_suzanne-thompson.
291. Alec Stratford, "Reflections on the Truth and Reconciliation Commission, Part Two," Transforming Edmonton, City of Edmonton (May 22, 2014). transforming.edmonton.ca/reflections-on-the-truth-and-reconciliation-commission-part-two/. Stratford is a descendant of Rev. Samuel Trivett.

292. Bruce Francis Macdonald, "Lieutenant Charlotte 'Lottie' Urquhart: A Military Medal Nursing Sister's Story," First World War Veterans of Guysborough County, May 31, 2018. guysboroughgreatwarveterans.blogspot.com/2018/05/lieutenant-charlotte-lottie-urquharta.html.
293. When he joined the CEF, he claimed that he was born in 1885, but his birth record in the Nova Scotia Archives states that he was born in 1884.
294. "Niagara Cemetery Index," Niagara Peninsula Branch, Ontario Ancestors. niagara.ogs.on.ca/cemetery_index/?wpda_search_column_index_id=77316/.
295. *Nurses' Directory*, 1923–24, 35.
296. "Lance Corporal William Francis Splatt," Canadian Virtual War Memorial, Veterans Affairs Canada. veterans.gc.ca/en/remembrance/memorials/canadian-virtual-war-memorial/detail/1596213?William%20Francis%20Splatt/.

Bibliography

Abbott, Maude E. "Lectures on the History of Nursing: With Descriptive List of Lantern-Slides." *Canadian Nurse and Hospital Review* vol. 19 (January 1923): 24–26. canadian-nurse.com/viewdocument/january-1923; vol. 19 (February 1923): 84–87. canadian-nurse.com/viewdocument/february-1923; vol. 19 (March 1923): 147–51. canadian-nurse.com/viewdocument/march-1923; vol. 19 (April 1923): 208–10. canadian-nurse.com/viewdocument/april-1923; vol. 19 (May 1923), 266–69. www.canadian-nurse.com/viewdocument/may-1923.

Adami, J. G. "The Enemy Air Raids upon Canadian Hospitals, May 1918: A Report to the DGMS Canadian Contingents." *Bulletin of the Canadian Army Medical Corps*, 1:5 (August 1918): 64–69. n2t.net/ark:/69429/m08w38051b68.

———. *War Story of the Canadian Army Medical Corps: The First Contingent*. Toronto: Published for the Canadian War Records Office by The Musson Book Company Ltd, 1918.

Adams, Annmarie. "Borrowed Buildings: Canada's Temporary Hospitals During World War I." *Canadian Bulletin of Medical History* 16:1 (Spring 1999): 25–48. doi.org/10.3138/cbmh.16.1.25.

Allard, Geneviève. "Caregiving on the Front: The Experience of Canadian Military Nurses During World War I." In *On All Frontiers: Four Centuries of Canadian Nursing*, edited by Christina Bates, Dianne Dodd, and Nicole Rousseau. Ottawa: University of Ottawa Press, 2005, 153–67.

———. "Des Anges blancs sur le front : L'Expérience de guerre des infirmières militaires canadiennes pendant la Première Guerre mondiale," *Bulletin d'histoire politique* 8:2–3 (Winter 2000): 119–33. doi.org/10.7202/1060202ar

Allemang, Margaret. "Canadian Nursing Sisters of World War I: Their Lives and Experiences in a Changing Society." *Proceedings of the Canadian Association for the History of Nursing Conferences, 1988 and 1990* (Calgary/Charlottetown: Canadian Association for the History of Nursing, 1988/90): 268–72.

Anon. "A Tale of a Casualty Clearing Station." *Canadian Nurse and Hospital Review*, vol. 13 (September 1917): 546–55. canadian-nurse.com/viewdocument/september-1917.

———. "Christmas in a Military Hospital." *Canadian Nurse and Hospital Review*, vol. 13 (December 1917): 753–54. canadian-nurse.com/viewdocument/december-1917.

———. "Dorothy Pearson Twist." Spanish Influenza in Victoria, Canada, 1918–1920: One City's Experience of the Great Pandemic. spanishfluvictoriabc.com/dorothy-pearson-twist/.

———. "French Flag Nursing Corps," *The British Journal of Nursing*, vol. 56 (January 1916): 18–27. rcnarchive.rcn.org.uk/volumes/56.

———. "Gone But Not Forgotten—Part 2: Sister Nurse Florence Louisa MacInnes and the Great War," *Halifax Blogs: Local History* (blog), Halifax Public Libraries, November 7, 2023. halifaxpubliclibraries.ca/blogs/post/gone-but-not-forgotten-part-2-sister-nurse-florence-louisa-macinnes-and-the-great-war/.

———. "J. R. M. Collie, MD, CM, MRCS, LRCP," *British Medical Journal* vol. 1 (1967): 369. doi.org/10.1136/bmj.1.5536.369.

———. "The Clayton Convalescent Home," *Canadian Medical Association Journal* vol. 6:10 (1916): 925–26. pmc.ncbi.nlm.nih.gov/articles/PMC1584771/.

———. "Experiences of a Canadian Nurse in France." *Canadian Nurse and Hospital Review* vol. 11 (May 1915): 258–61. canadian-nurse.com/viewdocument/may-1915.

———. "Voluntary Aid Detachment." Revised by Jenny Higgins, April 2015. In *Newfoundland & Labrador in the First World War*. Newfoundland and Labrador Heritage Web Site. heritage.nf.ca/first-world-war/articles/voluntary-aid-detachment.php.

———. "A History of the Boston Floating Hospital." *Pediatrics* 19:4 (1957): 629–38. doi.org/10.1542/peds.19.4.629.

Armstrong, John Griffith. *The Halifax Explosion and the Royal Canadian Navy: Inquiry and Intrigue*. Vancouver: UBC Press, 2002.

Arnold, Gertrude. "A Blighty Christmas: How Yuletide Was Spent Under the Red Cross." *Maclean's* vol. 32 (December 1919): 29–30, 79. archive.org/details/Macleans-Magazine-1919-12-01/page/n10/mode/1up/.

———. *Sister Anne! Sister Anne!* Toronto: McClelland & Stewart, c. 1919.

———. "The Search for Missing Men and Other Stories of a Canadian V.A.D." *Maclean's* vol. 32 (November 1919): 27–28, 75–79. archive.org/details/Macleans-Magazine-1919-11-01/page/n9/mode/1up/.

Attrill, Alfreda Jenness. "The Silent Ward." *Memoirs* (blog), *Legion Magazine*, March 5, 2017. legionmagazine.com/en/the-silent-ward/.

Baden-Powell, Olave. *Window on My Heart*. London: Hodder & Stoughton, 1973.

Beck, Boyde and Adele Townshend. "The Island's Florence Nightingale." *The Island Magazine* vol. 34 (Fall/Winter 1993): 1–6. islandarchives.ca/islandora/object/vre:islemag-batch2-449/.

Beckett, Andrew and Edward J. Harvey. "No 3 Canadian General Hospital (McGill) in the Great War: Service and Sacrifice," *Canadian Journal of Surgery* 61:1 (February 2018): 8–12. doi.org/10.1503/cjs.012717.

Bell, F. McKelvey. *A Romance of the Halifax Disaster*. Halifax: Royal Print & Litho, 1918.

——— *The First Canadians in France: The Chronicle of a Military Hospital in the War Zone*. New York: George H. Doran, 1917.

Bentley, Hannah. "Queen Alexandra's Imperial Military Nursing Service: A Study of Female Active Service During the First World War," Unpublished doctoral thesis, University of East Anglia, 2021. ueaeprints.uea.ac.uk/id/eprint/85348.

Bernier, Jean-Robert and Vivian C. McAlister. "The Canadian Army Medical Corps Affair of 1916 and Surgeon General Guy Carleton Jones," *Canadian Journal of Surgery* 61:2 (April 2018): 85–87. doi.org/10.1503/cjs.003818.

Boileau, John. *6/12/17: The Halifax Explosion*. Lunenburg: MacIntyre-Purcell Publishing, 2017.

Boylston, Helen Dore. *Sister: The War Diary of a Nurse*. New York: Ives Washburn, 1927.

Brookes, Alan A. "The Provincials by Albert J. Kennedy," *Acadiensis* 4:2 (1975): 85–101. jstor.org/stable/30302497.

Bruce, Constance. *Humour in Tragedy: Hospital Life Behind 3 Fronts by a Canadian Nursing Sister*. London: Skeffington & Son, 1918.

Burpee, Lawrence J. "The Canadian Medical Corps." Chap. 3 in *Canada in the Great World War*, vol. 6. Toronto: United Publishers of Canada, 1921.

Cahill, Barry. "Stewart, John (1848–1933)." *Dictionary of Canadian Biography*, vol. 16, University of Toronto/Université Laval, 2003–. biographi.ca/en/bio/stewart_john_1848_1933_16E.html.

C.A.M.C., Nursing Sister [pseud.]. "Military Nursing." *Canadian Nurse and Hospital Review*, vol. 13 (August 1917): 482–90. canadian-nurse.com/viewdocument/august-1917.

Cameron, James D. *For the People: A History of St Francis Xavier University*. Montreal & Kingston: McGill-Queen's University Press, 1966.

Cameron, James M. *Pictonians in Arms: A Military History of Pictou County, Nova Scotia*. Published by the author through The University of New Brunswick, 1969.

Carter, Joan. *Tears, Trials and Triumphs: A History of the Victoria General Hospital School of Nursing, 1891–1995*. Glen Margaret Publishing, 2005.

Carveth, Berta. "Diary of a Canadian Nurse Unit Four." In *We Wasn't Pals: Canadian Poetry and Prose of the First World War*, edited by Barry Callaghan and Bruce Meyer. Toronto: Exile Editions, 2001: 30–32.

Church, Haley. "Compassion Under Fire." *Mount Carmel Register*, December 16, 2016. newspapers.com/article/mount-carmel-register-bellenden-seymour/39702562/.

C. I. S., Nursing Sister [pseud.]. "Hospital Ship Life in the Mediterranean." *Canadian Nurse and Hospital Review* vol. 18 (January 1922): 29–34. canadian-nurse.com/viewdocument/january-1922.

Clint, Mabel B. "Le Touquet." *Canadian Nurse and Hospital Review* vol.11 (May 1915): 266–68. canadian-nurse.com/viewdocument/may-1915.

——— *Our Bit: Memories of War Service by a Canadian Nursing-Sister.* Montreal: Barwick, 1934: 110–19. Extract reprinted in *The War Diary of Clare Gass*, edited by Susan Mann. Montreal & Kingston: McGill-Queen's University Press, 2000: 249–58.

Cluett, Frances. *Your Daughter Fanny: The War Letters of Frances Cluett, VAD.* Edited by Bill Rompkey and Bert Riggs. St John's, NL: Flanker Press, 2006.

Collis, Elsie Dorothy. *Excerpts from Nursing Sister Elsie Collis' First World War Diary: A 1911 Graduate from Victoria's Royal Jubilee Hospital Training School.* Edited by Anne Pearson. Victoria, BC: Don & Anne Pearson, 1999.

Cook, Tim. "From the Great War to the Pandemic, Doctors and Nurses Have Always Carried a Heavy Burden," *The Globe and Mail*, September 15, 2022. theglobeandmail.com/opinion/article-a-long-continuum-of-caregivers-from-both-world-wars-to-the-present-day/.

Cook, Tim and J. L. Granatstein, eds., *Canada 1919: A Nation Shaped by War.* Vancouver: UBC Press, 2020.

Coombs, Howard G. "A Uniquely Canadian Military Moment: Sam Hughes and the No 7 General Hospital, 1915–1916," *Canadian Journal of Surgery* 60:4 (August 2017): 224–27. doi.org/10.1503/cjs.008717.

Cotton, Dorothy M. "A Word Picture of the Anglo-Russian Hospital, Petrograd." *The Canadian Nurse*, vol. 22 (September 1926): 486–88. canadian-nurse.com/viewdocument/september-1926.

———. "Balalaikas and Bandages." *Legion Magazine* vol. 62:5 (November 1987): 18–20.

Creed, Catherine, ed. "Flora H. Wylie." *Whose Debtors We Are. Niagara Historical Society* vol. 34 (1923): 73–84. notlmuseum.ca/research/society-publications?page=2.

Cushing, Harvey. *From A Surgeon's Journal 1915–1918.* London: Constable, 1936.

Delano, Jane A. "The Red Cross." *American Journal of Nursing*, 18:2 (November 1917): 124. journals.lww.com/ajnonline/citation/1917/11000/in_charge_of.12.aspx.

Dewar, Katherine. *Those Splendid Girls: The Heroic Service of Prince Edward Island Nurses in the Great War, 1914–1918*. Charlottetown: Island Studies Press, 2014.

Dodd, Dianne. "Canadian Military Nurse Deaths in the First World War." *Canadian Bulletin of Medical History* vol. 34:2 (September 2017): 327–63. doi.org/10.3138/cbmh.34.2.131-30072014.

———. "Local Markers: Canada's First World War Military Nurse Casualties." *Canadian Journal of Health History* vol. 39:2 (September 2022): 235–80. doi.org/10.3138/cjhh.2022-553-122021.

Drake, Harriet. *World War I Letters and Newspaper Clippings of Nursing Sister Harriet Drake*. Edited by Martha E. McKenna. Published by editor, 2007.

Drummond, Albert William. *Rhymes of a Hut-Dweller*. Published by author, [1918].

Duffus, Maureen. *Battlefront Nurses of WWI: The Canadian Army Medical Corps in England, France and Salonika, 1914–1919*. Victoria, BC: Town and Gown Press, 2009.

Duley, Margot I. "Nurse Martha Isabel Loder (1884–1963) and the Great War: From Snook's Harbour to the Somme," *Newfoundland Quarterly* vol. 108:3 (Winter 2015–16): 46–53. collections.mun.ca/digital/collection/quarterly/id/48435/rec/425.

Elliott, Wendy. "Nova Scotian Nurses Among the Unsung Heroes of the First World War," *Halifax Chronicle Herald*, October 2, 2014. Last updated September 30, 2017. saltwire.com/atlantic-canada/federal-election/nova-scotian-nurses-among-the-unsung-heroes-of-the-first-world-war-51724.

Fetherstonhaugh, Robert Collier. *No 3 Canadian General Hospital (McGill) 1914–1919*. Montreal: Gazette Printing Company, 1928.

Ford, Megan. "Focus: A Brief History of Men in Nursing." *Nursing Times*, March 6, 2019. nursingtimes.net/research-and-innovation/focus-a-brief-history-of-men-in-nursing-06-03-2019/.

Fowlds, Helen. "Gals at M." In *The Book of War Letters: 100 Years of Private Canadian Correspondence*. Edited by Paul and Audrey Grescoe. Toronto: MacFarlane, Walter & Ross, 2003: 100–03.

Fowler, T. Robert. "The Canadian Nursing Service and the British War Office: The Debate Over Awarding the Military Cross, 1918." *Canadian Military History* vol. 14:4 (2005): 31–42. scholars.wlu.ca/cmh/vol14/iss4/4/.

Fraser, Laura. "'Remember That I Love You': A Soldier's Letters to His Sweetheart." *CBC News*. newsinteractives.cbc.ca/longform/remember-that-i-love-you-a-soldiers-letters-to-his-sweetheart/.

Glassford, Sarah. "'Marching as to War': The Canadian Red Cross Society, 1885–1939." PhD dissertation, York University, 2007. academia.edu/3356009/_Marching_as_to_War_The_Canadian_Red_Cross_Society_1885_1939_York_University_PhD_dissertation_2007.

———. *Mobilizing Mercy*. Montreal & Kingston: McGill-Queen's University Press, 2017.

——— and Amy J. Shaw, eds. *A Sisterhood of Suffering and Service: Women and Girls of Canada and Newfoundland During the First World War*. Vancouver: UBC Press, 2012.

———. "Soldiering On After the Armistice: Health, Work and Family in the Lives of Some Canadian Army Medical Corps Nurse Veterans." *Canadian Military History* vol. 32:1 (2023): 1–24. scholars.wlu.ca/cmh/vol32/iss1/21/.

Grant, Amy Gordon, ed. *Letters from Armageddon: A Collection Made During the World War*. Boston/New York: Houghton Mifflin, 1930.

Gunn, Jean. "The Services of Canadian Nurses and Voluntary Aids During the War," *The Canadian Nurse* vol. 15 (September 1919): 1975–79. canadian-nurse.com/viewdocument/september-1919.

Gunn, John N. *Historical Records of Number 8 Canadian Field Ambulance: Canada, England, France, Belgium, 1915–1919*. Toronto: Ryerson Press, 1920.

Hacker, Carlotta. "The Bluebirds Who Went Over." *The Canadian Nurse* vol. 65 (November 1969): 31–34. canadian-nurse.com/viewdocument/november-1969.

Hallett, Christine E. "Portrayals of Suffering: Perceptions of Trauma in the Writings of First World War Nurses and Volunteers." *Canadian Bulletin of Medical History* vol. 27:1 (2010): 65–84. jstor.org/stable/45454731.

———. "Saving Lives on the Front Line." *History Today* vol. 67:7 (July 2017): 24–35. historytoday.com/archive/saving-lives-front-line/.

———. "The Personal Writings of First World War Nurses: A Study of the Interplay of Authorial Intention and Scholarly Interpretation." *Nursing Inquiry* vol. 14:4 (2007): 320–29. doi.org/10.1111/j.1440-1800.2007.00378.x.

———. *Veiled Warriors: Allied Nurses of the First World War*. Oxford University Press, 2014.

Hanna, Martha. "Behind the Lines: The 'War Books' of the Canadian Army Medical Corps, 1914–18." *Papers of the Bibliographical Society of Canada* vol. 53:2 (2016): 233–60. doi.org/10.33137/pbsc.v53i2.22555.

Hayes, Joseph. "Nova Scotia Medical Services in the Great War." In *Nova Scotia's Part in the Great War*, edited by M. S. Hunt. Halifax: The Nova Scotia Veteran Publishing, 1920:177–225.

Hebb, Ross, ed. *A Canadian Nurse in the Great War: The Diaries of Ruth Loggie, 1915–1916*. Halifax: Nimbus Publishing, 2021.

Hegan, Edith T. "The Russian Revolution from a Hospital Window." *Harper's Magazine* vol. 135:808 (September 1917): 555–61.

Higgins, Jenny. "Newfoundlanders and Labradorians in the First World War." Newfoundland and Labrador Heritage Web Site, April 2015. heritage.nf.ca/first-world-war/articles/nl-in-the-first-world-war.php.

Hogan, David B. "The Eventful History of the Number 9 Stationary Hospital (St Francis Xavier University), Canadian Army Medical Corps (1916–1920)," *Annals of the Royal College of Physicians and Surgeons of Canada* vol. 28:6 (September 1995): 354–58.

Hunt, M. S, ed. *Nova Scotia's Part in the Great War.* Halifax: The Nova Scotia Veteran Publishing, 1920.

Istil, Alexandra C. and Vivian C. McAlister. "Western University (No. 10 Canadian Stationary Hospital and No. 14 Canadian General Hospital): A Study of Medical Volunteerism in the First World War." *Canadian Journal of Surgery* vol. 59:6 (December 2016): 371–73. doi.org/10.1503/cjs.013716.

Johnson, Katherine Burger. "Called to Serve: American Nurses Go to War, 1914–1918." Paper 701, *Electronic Theses and Dissertations*, University of Louisville, 1993. doi.org/10.18297/etd/701.

Johnston, A. J. B. "Into the Great War: Katharine McLennan Goes Overseas, 1915–1919." In *The Island: New Perspectives on Cape Breton History 1713–1990*, edited by Kenneth Donovan. Sydney, NS: Acadiensis Press & UCCB Press, 1990: 129–44.

Jones, Peter. "A Thoroughly Cordial Relationship: A Narrative Account of the French Flag Nursing Corps 1914–19." *The Bulletin of the UK Association of the History of Nursing* vol. 6 (November 2017): 17–27. researchportal.lsbu.ac.uk/en/publications/a-thoroughly-cordial-relationship-a-narrative-accountof-the-frenc-3/.

Kelly, Alice. "'Can One Grow Used to Death?' Deathbed Scenes in Great War Nurses' Narratives." In *The Great War: From Memory to History*, edited by Kellen Kurchinski, Steve Marti, Alicia Robinet et al. Waterloo: Wilfrid Laurier University Press, 2015: 329–49.

Leddin, Desmond. *The No. 7 Canadian Stationary Hospital (Dalhousie University) in World War One.* Halifax: Red Barn Publishing, 2015.

——— and Paul Charlebois. "Treatment of Enemy Wounded: Evidence from the No. 7 Canadian Stationary Hospital (Dalhousie University)." *Canadian Journal of Surgery* vol. 60:1 (February 2017): 11–13. doi.org/10.1503/cjs.016716.

Leitch, M. Jessie. "Concerning 'Our First Glimpse of the Stars and Stripes in France': With Laval University Unit, Troyes, October, 1917." *Canadian Nurse and Hospital Review* vol. 17 (September 1921): 575–78. canadian-nurse.com/viewdocument/september-1921.

———. "Enemy Planes Were Observed Crossing the Coast." *Canadian Nurse and Hospital Review* vol. 18 (February 1922): 98–100. canadian-nurse.com/viewdocument/february-1922.

———. "En Route for France." *The Canadian Nurse* vol. 13 (December 1917): 748–50. canadian-nurse.com/viewdocument/december-1917.

Lindsay, Mabel. "A Tale of a Casualty Clearing Station." *Canadian Nurse and Hospital Review* vol. 13 (September 1917): 546–55. canadian-nurse.com/viewdocument/september-1917.

——— "Experiences of a Canadian Nurse in France." *The Canadian Nurse* vol. 11 (May 1915): 258–61. canadian-nurse.com/viewdocument/may-1915.

Lucas Rutherford, Mabel (Gertrude). "Canadian Nursing Sisters Are Always First Class." In *Voice of the Pioneer, vol. 2*, interviewed by Bill McNeil. Toronto: Macmillan (1984): 117–22.

——— "Sister Mabel Lucas—France, Gallipoli, Salonika, England, and Home." In *Seventy Years after 1914–1984*, edited by John Gardam. Stittsville, ON: Canada's Wings (1983): 46–49.

MacDonald, Bruce. "Sgt. Horace Goddard MacMillan: A 'Stationary Hospital' Soldier's Story." *First World War Veterans of Guysborough County*, May 30, 2013. guysboroughgreatwarveterans.blogspot.com/2013/05/sgt-horace-goddard-macmillan-stationary.html.

Macdonald, Clyde F. *Faithful Services in WWI and WWII: Veterans of Sunny Brae, Pictou County.* New Glasgow, NS: Pictou County Roots Society, 2001.

MacDonald, Hilda and Helen Kendall. "World War One Continues: Nursing-Sisters in England and France." *Cape Breton's Magazine* vol. 34 (August 1983): 1–7.

MacDonald, Katherine. "A Nursing Sister Near the Front, May 1918." In *Battle Lines: Eyewitness Accounts from Canada's Military History*, edited by J. L. Granatstein and Norman Hillmer. Toronto: Thomas Allen (2004): 191–92.

MacDonald, Laura M. *Curse of the Narrows: The Halifax Explosion 1917*. New York: Walker & Company, 2005.

Macdonald, Lyn. *The Roses of No Man's Land*. London: Michael Joseph, 1980.

Mackenzie, John Joseph. *Number 4 Canadian Hospital: The Letters of Professor J. J. Mackenzie from the Salonika Front*. Toronto: Macmillan, 1933.

MacLatchy, Katherine Osborne. "No. 3 Canadian General Hospital: Sailed from Montreal on the Metagama, May 6, 1915." *The Canadian Nurse* vol. 18 (July 1922): 414–18. canadian-nurse.com/viewdocument/july-1922. Reprinted as "Matron MacLatchy's Recollections." In *The War Diary of Clare Gass, 1915–1918*, edited by Susan Mann. Montreal & Kingston: McGill-Queen's University Press (2004): 243–7.

MacLeod, Alan Livingstone. "Catherine MacLean's War." Flickr Collections. Uploaded in 2010. flickr.com/photos/bigadore/collections/72157681517305405/.

Macleod, Jenny. *Gallipoli*, Great Battles. Oxford University Press, 2015.

Macphail, Andrew. *Official History of the Canadian Forces in the Great War 1914–19: The Medical Service*. Ottawa: F. A. Acland, King's Printer, 1925.

Mann, Susan. *Margaret Macdonald: Imperial Daughter*. Montreal & Kingston: McGill-Queen's Press, 2005.

———. "Where Have All the Bluebirds Gone? On the Trail of Canada's Military Nurses, 1914–1918." *Atlantis*, 26:1 (Fall/Winter 2001): 35–43. atlantisjournal.ca/index.php/atlantis/en/article/view/1498.

Marble, Dr. Allan. "Halifax Was Plunged into Gloom: The Impact of the Spanish Influenza Pandemic on Nova Scotia." *Journal of the Royal Nova Scotia Historical Society* vol. 22 (2019): 8–31.

Marquis, T. G. "First Canadian Unit in France." *Canada in the Great World War, Volume 2, Days of Preparation*. Toronto: United Publishers of Canada (1921): 299–304.

Matheson, Scott. "In the Dust You Will Prevail: The Mobilization of Acadia, Dalhousie, Mount Allison, and St. Francis Xavier Universities, 1914–1918." MA thesis, Halifax: Saint Mary's University, September 1, 2010. library2.smu.ca/handle/01/23728.

May, Robyn-Rose. *Bluebirds at War: Canada's Fallen Nursing Sisters of the First World War*. Toronto: Double Dagger Books, 2023.

McCarthy, Ethel M. *Report on the Work of the CAMC Nursing Service with the BEF in France. Great War Accounts: Canadian Nurses*, Scarlett Finders, copyright by The National Archives WO222/2134. scarletfinders.co.uk/20.html.

McGowan, Mark G. "Harvesting the 'Red Vineyard': Catholic Religious Culture in the Canadian Expeditionary Force 1914–1919." *Canadian Catholic Historical Association Historical Studies* vol. 64 (1998), 51–2, 61–64. cchahistory.ca/journal/CCHA1998/McGowan.htm.

McKenzie, Andrea. "'Our Common Colonial Voices': Canadian Nurses, Patient Relationships, and Nation on Lemnos." In *Other Fronts, Other Wars?: First World War Studies on the Eve of the Centennial*, History of Warfare, Volume 100, edited by Joachim Bürgschwentner, Matthias Egger and Gunda Barth-Scalmani. Leiden, The Netherlands: Brill (2014): 92–123. doi.org/10.1163/9789004279513_006.

——— "The Battle to Care: Canadian Nurses in France and Gallipoli." In *Two Sides of the Same Bad Penny?: Gallipoli and the Western Front, a Comparison*, edited by Michael LoCicero. Warwick, UK: Helion (2018): 209–29.

——— ed. *War-Torn Exchanges: The Lives and Letters of Nursing Sisters Laura Holland and Mildred Forbes*. Vancouver: UBC Press, 2016.

McPherson, Kathryn. "Carving Out a Past: The Canadian Nurses' Association War Memorial." *Histoire sociale/Social History* vol. 29:58 (November 1996): 417–30. hssh.journals.yorku.ca/index.php/hssh/article/view/4762.

Medical Society of Nova Scotia. "Nurses' Directory: Registered Nurses in Nova Scotia 1923–1924." *The Nova Scotia Medical Bulletin* vol. 3 (March 1924): 32–35. dalspace.library.dal.ca/items/691eca52-ec43-49c0-bb5c-8b91c5facc0b.

———. "Registered Nurses of Nova Scotia 1927." *The Nova Scotia Medical Bulletin* vol. 6 (December 1927): 29–35. dalspace.library.dal.ca/items/1b9af1f3-3bf3-49f6-b5e8-8b5deaa46acf.

Montgomery, Jennifer Sue. "Sisters, Objects of Desire, or Barbarians: German Nurses in the First World War" Master's Thesis, University of Tennessee, 2013. trace.tennessee.edu/utk_gradthes/2439/.

Monture, Edith Anderson. "Diary of a War Nurse [Edith Anderson Monture]." Ed. Terrie L. Monture Wicks. 1996. Photocopy of unpublished typescript. Toronto: Modern Literature and Culture Research Centre. wardiaries.ca/s/operationcanada/page/charlotte-edith-monture.

Moore, Mary Macleod. "Canadian Women War Workers Overseas." *The Canadian Magazine* vol. 52 (January 1919): 735–51.

——— "Our Doctors and Nurses in War Time." *Saturday Night Magazine*, 4 May 1918.

Morin-Pelletier, Mélanie. "'At Peace with the Germans, but at War with the Germs': Canadian Nurse Veterans After the First World War." In *Canada 1919: A Nation Shaped by War*, edited by Tim Cook and J. L. Granatstein. Vancouver: UBC Press (2020): 197–203.

——— "Bâtisseuses de l'est : les vétéranes des Maritimes et la santé publique, 1919–1939." *Acadiensis* vol. 42:1 (Winter/Spring 2013): 127–49. journals.lib.unb.ca/index.php/Acadiensis/article/view/20292.

——— *Briser les ailes de l'ange : les infirmières militaires canadiennes (1914–1918)*. Montreal: Athéna Editions, 2006.

Morrison, Ethel. "On Active Service." *The Canadian Nurse* vol. 34:1 (1938): 35–36. canadian-nurse.com/viewdocument/january-1938.

Morton, Desmond. *When Your Number's Up: The Canadian Soldier in the First World War*. Toronto: Random House, 1993.

Morton, Desmond and Glenn Wright. *Winning the Second Battle: Canadian Veterans and the Return to Civilian Life 1915–1930*. University of Toronto Press, 1987. jstor.org/stable/10.3138/j.ctvcj2rnz.

Mossman, David. *Going Over: A Nova Scotian Soldier in World War I*. Lawrencetown Beach: Pottersfield Press, 2014.

Mowat, Wilhelmina. "White Veils, Brass Buttons and Me." In *The Military Nurses of Canada: Recollections of Canadian Military Nurses, Volume 2*, edited by E. A. Landells. White Rock, BC: Co-Publishing (c1999): 46–61.

Nasmith, George G. *On the Fringe of the Great Fight.* Toronto: McClelland, Goodchild & Stewart, 1917.

Newell, Margaret Leslie. "'Led by the Spirit of Humanity': Canadian Military Nursing, 1914–1929." Thesis, University of Ottawa, 1996. Masters Abstracts International, Vol. 35(06): 1777. dx.doi.org/10.20381/ruor-8193.

Nicholson, Gerald W. L. *Canada's Nursing Sisters.* Toronto: Samuel Stevens Hakkert, 1975.

Norris, Marjorie Barron. *Sister Heroines: The Roseate Glow of Wartime Nursing, 1914–1918.* Calgary: Bunker to Bunker Publishing, 2002.

Nova Scotia Museum. "Repaying Neighbourly Kindness: Nova Scotia Nurses Travel to Boston." Remembering the Forgotten Dead Virtual Exhibit, Department of Communities, Culture, Tourism and Heritage. museum.novascotia.ca/collections-research/virtual-exhibits/remembering-forgotten-dead/repaying-neighbourly-kindness.

Parker, Ellanore J. *The Flower of the Land: A Tapestry of the Great War.* Los Angeles: DeVorss, 1941.

———. *The Land Lay Waiting.* New York: Pageant, 1955.

Paluszkiewicz-Misiaczek, Magdalena. "'Notwithstanding Its Awfulness...I Couldn't Have Stayed Away': The Great War in the Eyes of Canadian Military Nurses Sophie Hoerner and Dorothy Cotton." In *Re-Imagining the First World War: New Perspectives in Anglophone Literature and Culture*, edited by Anna Branach-Kallas and Nelly Strehlau. Cambridge: Cambridge Scholars (2015): 314–29. ruj.uj.edu.pl/xmlui/handle/item/17760.

Pirie, A. H. *No. 3 Canadian General Hospital (McGill) in France (1915, 1916, 1917): with Views Illustrating Life and Scenes in the Hospital with a Short Description of Its Origin, Organisation and Progress.* Middlesbrough, UK: Hood, 1923.

Putnam, Eben, ed. *Report of the Commission on Massachusetts' Part in the World War, Volume 1.* Boston: Commonwealth of Massachusetts, 1931. familysearch.org/library/books/records/item/136917-report-of-the-commission-on-massachusetts-part-in-the-world-war-v-01?offset=1/.

Quiney, Linda J. "Assistant Angels: Canadian Voluntary Aid Detachment Nurses in the Great War." *Canadian Bulletin of Medical History* vol. 15:1 (1998): 189–206. doi.org/10.3138/cbmh.15.1.189.

———. "'Bravely and Loyally They Answered the Call': St John Ambulance, the Red Cross, and the Patriotic Service of Canadian Women During the Great War." *History of Intellectual Culture* vol. 5:1 (2005). journalhosting.ucalgary.ca/index.php/hic/article/view/68887.

———. "'Filling the Gaps': Canadian Voluntary Nurses, the 1917 Halifax Explosion, and the Influenza Epidemic of 1918." *Canadian Bulletin of Medical History* vol. 19:2 (2002): 351–74. doi.org/10.3138/cbmh.19.2.351.

———. "Gendering Patriotism: Canadian Volunteer Nurses as the Female 'Soldiers' of the Great War." In *A Sisterhood of Suffering and Service: Women and Girls of Canada and Newfoundland During the First World War*, edited by Sarah Glassford and Amy J. Shaw. Vancouver: UBC Press (2012): 103–25.

———. "'Sharing the Halo': Social and Professional Tensions in the Work of World War I Canadian Volunteer Nurses." *Journal of the Canadian Historical Association* vol. 9:1 (1998): 105–24. doi.org/10.7202/030494ar.

———. *This Small Army of Women: Canadian Volunteer Nurses and the First World War.* Vancouver: UBC Press, 2018.

Quinn, Shawna M. *Agnes Warner and the Nursing Sisters of the Great War.* Fredericton: Goose Lane Editions, 2010.

Raddall, Thomas H. *In My Time: A Memoir.* Toronto: McClelland and Stewart, 1976.

Rawling, William. *Death Their Enemy: Canadian Medical Practitioners and War.* Ottawa: Privately published, 2001.

Rolls, Vanessa Childs. "How the Workers Took Control of Health Care in Glace Bay." *Cape Breton Post,* March 31, 2017. Last updated October 2, 2017. saltwire.com/cape-breton/opinion/column-how-the-workers-took-control-of-health-care-in-glace-bay-21479/.

Rosenthal, Lyndsay. "Venus in the Trenches: The Treatment of Venereal Disease in the Canadian Expeditionary Force, 1914–1919." *Theses and Dissertations (Comprehensive).* 2107. (2018). scholars.wlu.ca/etd/2107.

Rudolf, R. D. "Boulogne in War Time." *Canadian Medical Association Journal* vol. 5:3 (March 1915): 255–59. pmc.ncbi.nlm.nih.gov/articles/PMC1487140/.

Satchell, Patricia. "MacIntosh Rebecca." *Bodelwyddan Memorial,* Flintshire War Memorials. flintshirewarmemorials.com/memorials/bodelwyddan-memorial/canadians-2/macintosh-rebecca/.

Smith, Thomas Brenton. "Clearing: The Tale of the First Canadian Casualty Clearing Station BEF, 1914–1919." Unpublished, Dalhousie University Archives.

Spicer, Stanley T. *Maritimers Ashore & Afloat: Interesting People, Places and Events Related to the Bay of Fundy and Its Rivers.* Hantsport: Lancelot Press, 1993.

Stephens, Gloria (Webb). "1917–The Halifax Explosion and the VG Hospital." Nova Scotia Museum of Health Care, Association of Health Sciences Archives and Museums of Nova Scotia. novascotiamuseumofhealthcare.ca/resources/articles/.

———. *Remembering Nurses Who Served.* Halifax: MacKenzie Publishing, 2020.

Stewart, Ronald D. "The Long Trail Winding." *VoxMeDal* (Spring 2008): 21–22. cdn.dal.ca/content/dam/dalhousie/pdf/faculty/medicine/departments/core-units/DMAA/voxmedal/vox_spring08.pdf.

Stirling, Terry Bishop. "'Such Sights One Will Never Forget': Newfoundland Women and Overseas Nursing in the First World War." In *A Sisterhood of Suffering and Service: Women and Girls of Canada and Newfoundland During the First World War*, edited by Sarah Glassford and Amy J. Shaw. Vancouver: UBC Press (2012): 126–47.

Stuart, Meryn. "Social Sisters: A Feminist Analysis of the Discourses of Canadian Military Nurse Helen Fowlds, 1915–18." In *Place and Practice in Canadian Nursing History*, edited by Jayne Elliott, Meryn Stuart, and Cynthia Toman. Vancouver: UBC Press (2008): 25–39.

Summers, Anne. "Women as Voluntary and Professional Military Nurses in Great Britain 1854–1914." PhD Thesis, Open University, 1985. doi.org/10.21954/ou.ro.0000de51.

Tennyson, Brian Douglas. *Canada's Great War, 1914–1918: How Canada Helped Save the British Empire and Became a North American Nation.* Lanham: Roman & Littlefield, 2015.

———. *Nova Scotia at War 1914–1919.* Halifax: Nimbus, 2017.

———. *The Canadian Experience of the Great War: A Guide to Memoirs.* Lanham: Scarecrow Press, 2013.

Thornhill, Bonnie and W. James MacDonald, eds, *In the Morning: Biographical Sketches of the Veterans of Victoria County, Cape Breton, That Served in Both World Wars.* Sydney: UCCB Press, 1999.

Toman, Cynthia. "'A Loyal Body of Empire Citizens': Military Nurses and Identity at Lemnos and Salonika, 1915–17." In *Place and Practice in Canadian Nursing History*, edited by Jayne Elliott, Meryn Stuart, and Cynthia Toman. Vancouver: UBC Press (2008):8–24.

———. "Georgina Fane Pope." *The Canadian Encyclopedia*, Historica Canada. Published December 13, 2007. Last edited March 7, 2016. thecanadianencyclopedia.ca/en/article/georgina-fane-pope/.

———. "'Help Us, Serve England': First World War Military Nursing and National Identities." *Canadian Bulletin of Medical History* vol. 30:1 (2013): 143–66. doi.org/10.3138/cbmh.30.1.143.

———. *Sister Soldiers of the Great War: The Nurses of the Canadian Army Medical Corps.* Vancouver: UBC Press, 2016.

Tucker, Gilbert Norman. *The Naval Service of Canada: Its Official History.* Ottawa: King's Printer, 1962.

Tylee, Claire M. *The Great War and Women's Consciousness: Images of Militarism and Womanhood in Women's Writings.* Iowa City: University of Iowa Press, 1990.

Veterans Affairs Canada. *Canada's Nursing Sisters.* Charlottetown, PEI: Veterans Affairs Canada, 2005.

Wagner, Suzanna. "Many Places, Many Problems: Canadian First World War Military Nursing Sisters in the Mediterranean." Master's Thesis, University of Alberta, 2020. doi.org/10.7939/r3-56vz-9t73.

Warner, Agnes (Louise). *My Beloved Poilus.* Saint John, NB: Barnes, 1917. Reprinted as *Nurse at the Trenches: Letters Home from a WWI Nurse.* Burgess Hill, UK: Diggory Press, 2005.

White, James F. E. *The Garrison Response to the Halifax Disaster, 6 December 1917.* Halifax Defence Complex, Parks Canada, 2014.

Wells, Jeannette. "I Was a V.A.D." Interviewed by Iris Power. *Atlantic Guardian* vol. 11:5 (July 1954): 26–30. collections.mun.ca/u?/guardian,4250.

Wilkinson, Maude. "Four Score and Ten." *The Canadian Nurse* vol. 73 (October 1977): 26–29. canadian-nurse.com/viewdocument/october-1977. (November 1977): 14–22. canadian-nurse.com/viewdocument/november-1977 (December 1977): 16–23. canadian-nurse.com/viewdocument/december-1977. Expanded version published as *Four Score and Ten: Memoirs of a Canadian Nurse.* Brampton, ON: M.M. Armstrong, 2003.

Williams, Fred and Dr. Ken Murray. *To Heal Sometimes, to Comfort Always: A History of the Care of the Sick North of Smokey.* Ingonish: Buchanan Memorial Hospital, 1993.

Williams, John. *The Other Battleground: The Home Fronts: Britain, France and Germany, 1914–18.* Chicago: Henry Regnery, 1972.

Wilson-Simmie, Katherine M. *Lights Out! The Memoir of Nursing Sister Kate Wilson, Canadian Army Medical Corps, 1915–1917.* Ottawa: CEF Books, 2004.

Wyman, Marlena. "Bluebird: Madeleine Jaffray." *The Prairie Line*, December 6, 2018. theprairieline.wordpress.com/2018/12/06/bluebird-madeleine-jaffray/.

Young, Frances. "The Halifax Disaster." *The Canadian Nurse* vol. 14 (January 1918): 797–9. canadian-nurse.com/viewdocument/january-1918.

Digital Sources

Wikipedia.org, "Canadian Nurses Who Died in World War I." en.wikipedia.org/wiki/List_of_Canadian_nurses_who_died_in_World_War_I.

First World War Veterans of Guysborough County. guysboroughgreatwarveterans.blogspot.com.

Lives of the First World War, "Bluebirds: Canadian Nurses of WWI." livesofthefirstworldwar.iwm.org.uk/community/2605/.

Index

Symbols

A

B

C

E

G

H

I

J

M

O

S

U

V

W

Y

Z